The Mighty Baby

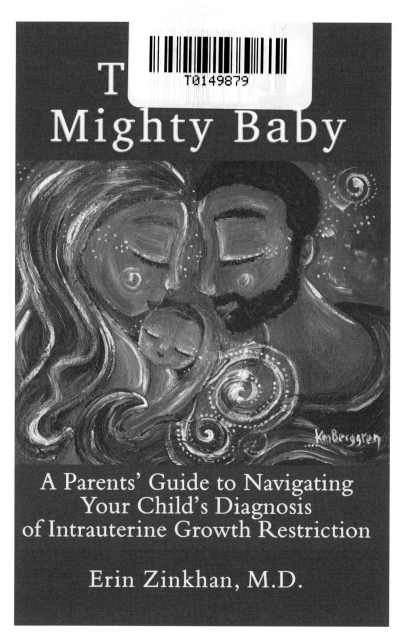

A Parents' Guide to Navigating Your Child's Diagnosis of Intrauterine Growth Restriction

Erin Zinkhan, M.D.

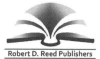

Robert D. Reed Publishers

Robert D. Reed Publishers • Bandon, OR

Robert D. Reed Publishers
P.O. Box 1992
Bandon, OR 97411
Phone: 541-347-9882; Fax: -9883
E-mail: 4bobreed@msn.com
Website: www.rdrpublishers.com

Editor: Cleone Reed
Designer: Amy Cole
Cover: Cleone Reed
Cover Artwork: *Catching My Angel* © Katie m. Berggren

Soft Cover ISBN: 978-1-944297-97-8
EBook ISBN: 978-1-944297-98-5

Library of Congress Control Number: 2021934559

Designed and Formatted in the United States of America

Parent's stories freely provided and permission granted to publish them in this book.

Praise for the book

"I've read through the manuscript—wow! I found it both engaging and informative and I bet other parents will as well. I was also in tears at parts."

"I read the whole thing and loved it. I think it's very informative and will be a powerful tool for parents with growth-restricted babies. I really liked reading the parents' stories, too."

"I would honestly have found this book to be very useful after my son's birth; so much of it makes more sense now, in retrospect."

"I just read the book and it's great! I'd also love to give a thanks for including a story of infant loss. Too often these stories are not given a voice in hopes of not scaring others. It is very meaningful to have one in the book."

Acknowledgments

I am extremely honored to have had the privilege to work with Eliana, Laura, Alex, Catie, Michele, Sandra, Hilarie, Colby, Jen, Meagan, and their families who have contributed to this book in tremendous ways. I thank them from the depths of my heart for their honesty and vulnerability in sharing their stories and providing feedback about this book.

I am particularly grateful to my medical illustrator, Megan Rojas, and to the physicians who have reviewed this book to ensure accuracy. These physicians are Dr. Jeanette Carpenter in Maternal-Fetal Medicine, Dr. Ryann Bierer in Neonatology and Palliative Care, and Dr. George Zinkhan in Neurology.

TINY BUT MIGHTY BABY

Contents

ACKNOWLEDGMENTS v

INTRODUCTION 1

CHAPTER 1: What Is Growth Restriction? 5

CHAPTER 2: How Is Growth Restriction
      Diagnosed and Managed during Pregnancy? 29

CHAPTER 3: What Are Effects of Growth
      Restriction in Full-term Newborns? 45

CHAPTER 4: What Are Effects of Growth
      Restriction in Premature Newborns? 65

CHAPTER 5: How Does Growth Restriction
      Impact Health in Childhood through Adulthood? ... 95

CONCLUSION 117

APPENDIX 1: Resources for Families 119

APPENDIX 2: Tenth Percentile Weight for
      Each Gestational Age 121

APPENDIX 3: IUGR and NICU Glossary 125

ABOUT THE AUTHOR 131

Introduction

You are probably reading this book because your baby, or the baby of a loved one, has been diagnosed with intrauterine growth restriction. You probably have many questions. The good news is that most babies with growth restriction, especially those born at or near full-term, do very well in infancy and through adulthood. More good news is that you are not alone. Approximately one in ten babies are diagnosed with growth restriction, so hundreds of thousands of parents face this diagnosis each year in the United States alone. I hope this book can help you understand what growth restriction means, answer many of your questions, and help you feel confident about caring for your tiny but mighty baby.

I have spent my career in academic Neonatology studying the long-term health effects of growth restriction and have published many articles on the topic. The idea of writing a book about growth restriction for families had not crossed my mind, though, until a few insightful parents prompted me. The idea for this book started when I was sitting at a baby's bedside in the Neonatal Intensive Care Unit (NICU). I was educating the baby's parents about growth restriction and the role it plays in their baby's health. They had not heard of growth restriction before their baby came under my care. Our discussion covered everything from how growth restriction is diagnosed to what complications their baby might face in the NICU and later in life. During our discussion, the mother was holding a book about the NICU in her hands, and it dawned on me that parents might really benefit from a book about growth restriction.

The idea remained in the back of mind for several months until I met another set of parents in a social setting outside of the hospital. The parents remembered me because I had taken care of their daughter in the NICU. Their daughter's care was complicated by growth restriction, and as we talked, I asked them whether they might appreciate a book written for parents with growth-restricted babies. They, too, had read every book available to parents about the NICU and still thought that the diagnosis of growth restriction was difficult to understand and a bit scary. They both thought that a book dedicated to growth restriction would have been helpful while they were in the NICU. They contributed one of the stories to this book.

This book represents a true partnership between me as a neonatologist and the families that have contributed to it. I have had the privilege of working with many wonderful parents who have been willing to share their stories with me and with you. The stories are told in their own words with only light editing for clarity and privacy. This book also addresses questions raised by their experiences, in a question-and-answer format.

Their stories are personal and intimate. Please be aware that while many have happy endings, some involve sensitive and painful subjects, including miscarriage and infant loss. The vulnerability, emotion, and resilience that comes through in their stories is truly powerful and moving. I am grateful to these families for their generosity and honesty in sharing with us so that other families can better understand and navigate a diagnosis of intrauterine growth restriction. Except in the family stories, I have chosen to alternate the use of "she / her" pronouns with "he / him" pronouns by chapter when referring to the baby. I also use the terms "mother" and "father" to indicate the biological mother and biological father, as I often am referring to the sharing of genetic information.

A diagnosis of growth restriction can be confusing and frightening. Even though growth restriction is relatively common, most parents have never heard the term before. Many physicians do not understand how growth restriction can affect a baby's health throughout life. Explaining the diagnosis of growth restriction to friends and family can be even more challenging. If you are in this situation, I encourage you to give this book to your friends and family, and let it teach them how your tiny baby can grow up to be strong. You also can refer them to my blog at www.tinybutmightybaby.com to ask questions, find answers, or find updates on research about growth restriction. This book and the www.tinybutmightybaby.com website are intended solely for educational purposes. It cannot substitute for the advice, diagnosis, treatment, or supervision of a medical professional. Always discuss any specific health concerns or questions with your doctor. This book also reflects my own opinions about growth restriction and not that of any of my current or previous professional affiliations.

The best advice that I can give a parent trying to navigate a diagnosis of growth restriction is summed up by one of the parents who helped me with this book. She wrote:

"If we could share some advice: please do not let an IUGR diagnosis define your pregnancy. It is so easy for the endless doctors' appointments, terrifying Google searches, and sleepless nights to drain the joy out of what should be one of the most magical times of your life. Do everything you can to enjoy the times in between. Make sure to enjoy every kick, every ultrasound, every awkward encounter with a stranger who wants to feel your belly, and the infectious excitement from those around you. Take joy in the endless research needed to create the perfect registry, the long nights of decorating and painting the nursery of your dreams, and watching your partner fumble through the construction of the 'some assembly required' baby furniture. Because for each hard moment you have in your pregnancy, there are a million memories like these that far outweigh them."

CHAPTER 1

What Is Growth Restriction?

Most babies diagnosed with intrauterine growth restriction (IUGR) grow up to live full and healthy lives. The diagnosis of growth restriction, however, can increase the risk of certain health problems from birth throughout life. We will discuss the potential health risks that can be associated with intrauterine growth restriction later in this book, but first we need to talk about what intrauterine growth restriction is.

The technical definition of intrauterine growth restriction is the inability of a fetus to meet her growth potential. If this definition is confusing to you, then you are not alone. I remember having difficulty understanding this term when I was in my pediatrics residency, and I had already finished medical school! To this day I still am asked by physicians at all levels of training how to define growth restriction, and most physicians who take care of adults do not know that growth restriction may impact health throughout life. To make matters more complicated, you may hear your obstetrician or your baby's pediatrician only use the term, "IUGR," which is the abbreviation for intrauterine growth restriction. Further, physicians and researchers sometimes use the term "fetal growth restriction" instead of "intrauterine growth restriction." I have chosen to use the more traditional term "intrauterine growth restriction," which I often will shorten to "growth restriction" in this book.

I think the best definition of growth restriction is simply this: the baby is smaller than she should be. The hard part is knowing what a baby's growth "should be." Sometimes it may not be clear whether a baby has growth restriction. This lack of clarity about whether the baby has growth restriction may mean physicians are reluctant to make the diagnosis except in the most extreme cases. We will talk more about how physicians diagnose growth restriction in the next chapter.

Pediatricians use a formula based on the heights of the biological parents to calculate the expected range of a particular child's height, which is called the midparental height. The midparental height takes into account the heights of each biological parent and whether the child is a boy or a girl. A child who is shorter than her expected height range may have growth that is less than it should be. To understand what a baby's growth should be, we need to understand how growth is determined. Genes determine growth potential. For example, if a baby has two tall biological parents, we expect the baby to be tall because she gets one tall gene from her father and one tall gene from her mother. But if she is shorter and weighs less than expected, then she may not have reached her growth potential and may be growth restricted (**Figure 1**).

On the other hand, if a baby has two short biological parents, we expect that she will be short because she gets one short gene from her father and one from her mother. If the baby is also short, it is probably normal for her (**Figure 1**). However, sometimes when a short baby is born to two short parents, she may be growth restricted.

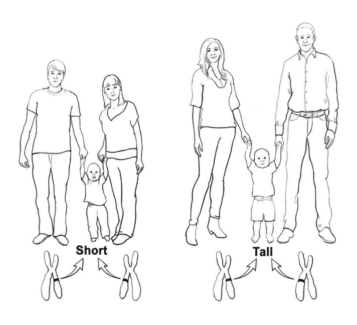

Tall parents will pass along genes to their children that will make them tall. Short parents will pass along genes to their children to make them short.

Figure 1

There is a difference between growth restriction and "small for gestational age" (SGA). The definition of SGA is defined solely by body weight, and simply means that the baby's birth weight is lower than the tenth percentile for gestational age. Lower than the tenth percentile means that the baby's weight is less than the weight of nine out of every ten babies born at the same gestational age. Some of the babies that are diagnosed as SGA are completely healthy. These babies may be small because their biological parents are small, and we expect the baby to be small. On the other hand, some SGA babies are also growth restricted. An example would be when a baby is born to tall biological parents, but the baby is small. The most challenging case of growth restriction for physicians to identify is when the baby's weight is greater than the tenth percentile. This baby may have growth restriction even though she is not SGA. For example, if a baby born to two very tall parents is at the twentieth percentile for weight and length, this baby may have growth restriction even though she is not SGA.

The definition that obstetricians and Maternal Fetal Medicine physicians use for growth restriction is different than the one used by pediatricians and neonatologists. While the definition of SGA is the same for these physicians, for obstetricians, growth restriction is diagnosed before birth in a fetus whose weight is estimated by ultrasound to be less than the tenth percentile for gestational age. Pediatricians and neonatologists may use fetal ultrasounds and a baby's physical features after birth to diagnose a baby with growth restriction. For the purposes of this book, we will use the pediatricians' and neonatologists' definition of growth restriction.

There are many reasons why a baby may be smaller than she should be. These reasons can be broken down into three general categories: infectious, environmental, and genetic/syndromic/structural (**Figure 2**).

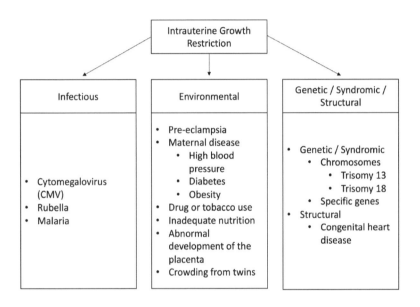

Causes of intrauterine growth restriction.

Figure 2

Infectious causes are problems caused by viruses, bacteria, or other organisms. Environmental causes are problems with the environment in the womb. Genetic causes are problems caused by genes inherited from biological parents. A syndrome is a collection of findings that are commonly found in people with a specific genetic disorder, although sometimes the exact change to the genes is not known. Structural changes are problems in how specific parts of the body, such as the heart, develop. These changes can impact how the whole body grows.

Sometimes physicians and researchers use different categories to describe the reasons why a baby is smaller than she should be. These other categories may be fetal (related to the baby), placental (related to the placenta), and maternal (related to the mother). Fetal causes include problems with the genes, structural changes to the body, and infections. Placental causes occur when the placenta develops abnormally or when a baby is sharing the placenta with a twin. Maternal causes occur when maternal health conditions are present.

The specific categories are not as important as identifying the underlying cause of growth restriction because the cause may influence the health challenges that the baby may have after birth or later in life. For the purposes of this book, we will use the categories of genetic, infectious, and environmental to facilitate understanding of the many potential causes of growth restriction. We will focus primarily on the effects of growth restriction from environmental causes because these are the most common causes in countries like the United States. But first we will discuss briefly the genetic and infectious causes of growth restriction. The health challenges that growth-restricted babies may face after birth are different depending on what caused the growth restriction. When growth restriction is caused by a genetic or infectious cause, the challenges these babies face are primarily due to the underlying genetic or infectious cause rather than due to growth restriction itself.

There are many genetic causes of growth restriction. One genetic cause of growth restriction is the baby having an extra chromosome. A chromosome is a large collection of genes. Humans have 23 pairs of chromosomes (**Figure 3**).

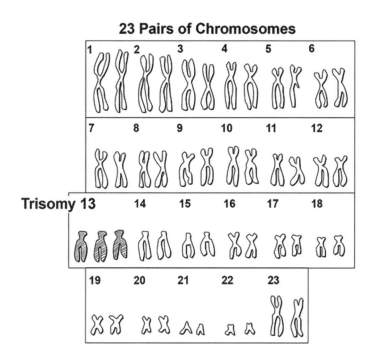

23 Pairs of Chromosomes

We each have 23 pairs of chromosomes. One chromosome from each pair comes from our mother and one from our father. Sometimes we get an extra chromosome from one of our parents. If the extra chromosome is the 13th chromosome, it causes a condition called trisomy 13.

Figure 3

11

We get 23 chromosomes from our biological father and 23 from our biological mother. Each chromosome is named after a number such as chromosome 1, chromosome 2, etc. If a person has an extra chromosome, then the condition the person has is named after the number of the extra chromosome. For example, trisomy 21, which is commonly known as Down syndrome, refers to a person having three copies of chromosome 21 instead of the usual two copies. Although trisomy 21 does not cause growth restriction necessarily, other syndromes with extra chromosomes often do, such as trisomy 13 and trisomy 18 **(Figure 3)**. Sometimes the specific genetic abnormality is not known, but the baby has features that suggest the baby may have a syndrome. The underlying genetic cause of Edwards syndrome is known to be an extra copy of chromosome 18, and one of the common findings in Edwards syndrome is growth restriction. There are many other genetic abnormalities that cause growth restriction. Genetic disorders and syndromes can be inherited from parent to child, or they can occur when there is a new change to the genes in the developing fetus.

Other structural conditions associated with growth restriction can occur without a clear genetic or infectious cause. One example is congenital heart disease, which is a problem with how the baby's heart formed. In a condition like this, the long-term health of the baby is influenced primarily by the underlying structural problem more than by growth restriction itself. For example, in a baby with both growth restriction and congenital heart disease, the congenital heart disease will have a significantly greater impact on the baby's health than the initial growth restriction. However, a baby that has congenital heart disease and does not have growth restriction generally will have a better outcome than a baby with both congenital heart disease and growth restriction.

Infections are the cause of impaired growth in about one in every ten to twenty cases of growth restriction. How the growth restriction happens depends on both the type of infection and when the infection occurs during pregnancy. One of the most common infectious causes of growth restriction globally is malaria. Fortunately, malaria is extremely uncommon in the United States. Bacteria may cause chorioamnionitis, which is inflammation of the placenta and amniotic fluid. This is called intrauterine inflammation or infection, or "Triple I." Although most bacteria are not specifically known to cause growth restriction, Triple I is associated with growth restriction. Some viruses also may cause growth restriction. Two of the most well-studied viruses that cause growth restriction are rubella and cytomegalovirus (CMV). Most pregnant women have been immunized against rubella and have had CMV in childhood, and thus are at low risk for these infections during pregnancy.

It is important to know that even though a mother and fetus may be infected with a virus, it does not mean that the virus always will cause problems. Sometimes the mother's body can control the infection without affecting the baby. Other times the infection occurs without the mother even knowing. CMV, for example, can cause cold-like or flu-like symptoms in a pregnant mother, or sometimes it can infect her without causing any symptoms at all. When an infection causes growth restriction, the short- and long-term health of the baby is influenced more by what causes the infection and when in pregnancy it happens than specifically by growth restriction.

The last category of causes of growth restriction is environmental. The fetal environment is the womb, the mother, and the mother's environment. Many environmental factors can decrease the delivery of nutrients and oxygen through the placenta to the fetus. The most common cause of growth restriction in developed countries is preeclampsia. Preeclampsia is a condition that only pregnant mothers can develop. Preeclampsia is most often diagnosed when a pregnant mother has high blood pressure and protein in the urine. In pregnancies affected by preeclampsia, the placenta often does not work as well and may cause the fetus to not get enough blood flow, nutrition, and oxygen. However, researchers are starting to learn that the connection between preeclampsia and growth restriction is probably more complicated.

Health conditions in the mother also may cause growth restriction in the fetus. High blood pressure, even without other signs of preeclampsia, can reduce the delivery of nutrients and oxygen to the fetus. Obesity and diabetes in pregnant mothers most often cause babies to be larger than normal but, in some cases, can cause growth restriction. When a fetus is larger than the 90th percentile (larger than nine of out every ten) of fetuses at a specific gestational age, the condition is called large for gestational age (LGA). Babies who are either growth restricted or large for gestational age have many of the same potential health risks later in life. We will discuss more about these potential life-long health risks later in this book.

Medications taken by the biological mother also can increase the risk that a fetus develops growth restriction. Certain anti-seizure medications and a certain blood clot prevention medication called warfarin can increase the risk of growth restriction. Reviewing your medications with your physician and, if needed, changing your medications may reduce the risk that your fetus will develop growth restriction.

Other environmental factors can cause growth restriction. Smoking, drinking alcohol, or using illicit drugs during pregnancy can not only cause growth restriction, but also expose the baby to toxic substances. While many women are motivated to quit smoking, drinking alcohol, or using illicit drugs during pregnancy for the health of their baby, pregnancy and having a newborn can be stressful, making it even harder to quit. Even if the mother does not smoke, the developing fetus and child may develop health problems due to exposure to second-hand smoke and third-hand smoke. Second-hand smoke exposure is exposure to tobacco smoke from other smokers even if the pregnant mother does not smoke. Third-hand smoke exposure is exposure to clothing, furniture, or the inside of a car, where a person has been smoking tobacco. To improve the health of the baby, it is important that pregnant women and their household members seek help from partners, friends, family, and professionals if needed to quit smoking, drinking alcohol, or using illicit drugs.

Sometimes growth restriction may be caused by an abnormal placenta. The placenta is the organ that attaches to the inside of the womb and provides nutrients and oxygen to the developing fetus through the umbilical cord (**Figure 4**). When the placenta is not formed correctly, the placenta

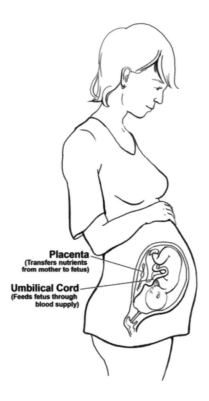

Placenta
(Transfers nutrients
from mother to fetus)

Umbilical Cord
(Feeds fetus through
blood supply)

*The placenta filters nutrients and oxygen from the mother's blood
and gives them to the fetus through the umbilical cord.*

Figure 4

may not provide enough nutrition for the fetus. Normally
the placenta grows fairly proportionately with the fetus so
that the placenta gets bigger as the fetus grows. Placentas
from pregnancies complicated by growth restriction are

typically smaller than normal. However, even a normally-sized placenta may not work normally. If the placenta does not grow well, the amount of nutrition that the baby needs may exceed what the placenta can provide. In other words, the fetus may "outgrow" the placenta.

Sometimes the umbilical cord may be attached in an abnormal position on the placenta, which impairs the ability of the placenta to get adequate nutrition to the fetus. Researchers are looking into the pathways that cause a placenta to develop abnormally and ways to help the placenta deliver proper nutrition to the fetus. Twins, triplets, and other multiple fetuses that share a placenta are more likely to have growth restriction. This predisposition can occur not only from crowding in the womb but also from unequal sharing of blood from the placenta. Unequal sharing of blood sometimes can be related to a condition called twin-to-twin transfusion syndrome, a condition where one fetus is significantly smaller than the other because she is "donating" blood to her twin. Up to one quarter of twins and more than half of triplets and quadruplets will have growth restriction.

Growth restriction from genetic, infectious, and environmental causes may cause symmetric or asymmetric growth restriction (**Figure 5**). Using ultrasound images before the baby is born or from measurements done by hospital staff after the baby is born, physicians can plot the baby's weight, length, and head circumference on a growth chart specific to the baby's gestational age at birth. If all the measurements are equally small, then the baby may be considered to have symmetric growth restriction. However, if the baby's weight is decreased more significantly than the length

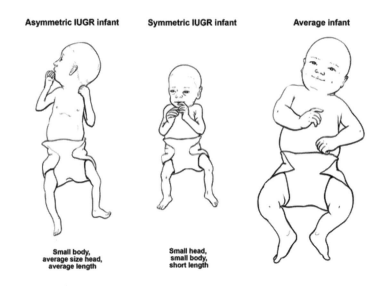

Asymmetric IUGR infant	Symmetric IUGR infant	Average infant
Small body, average size head, average length	Small head, small body, short length	

*Asymmetric growth restriction compared
with symmetric growth restriction.*

Figure 5

or head circumference are decreased, then the baby is considered to have asymmetric growth restriction. Obstetricians also may use ultrasound measurements to evaluate for the type of growth restriction a fetus has. If the size of the fetus's abdomen or stomach is decreased more significantly than the estimated weight of the fetus or length of the bones in the legs, then the fetus may be considered to have asymmetric growth restriction. Physicians use these categories to help determine what caused the growth restriction. For example, genetic or infectious causes of growth restriction often cause symmetric growth restriction, while preeclampsia often causes asymmetric growth restriction.

Asymmetric growth restriction usually occurs later during pregnancy than symmetric growth restriction. As noted, a common cause of asymmetric growth restriction is preeclampsia. Preeclampsia is diagnosed usually in the second half of pregnancy, but researchers have found small changes in the blood vessels of the placenta even in the first trimester in pregnancies before preeclampsia develops. These changes may limit how much nutrition and oxygen the fetus receives. As the fetus grows, she may need more nutrition than what the placenta can give her.

One way the fetus protects herself when she does not get enough nutrition is to change how the blood vessels in her body develop. She may redirect blood flow to her brain, giving the brain more nutrition and leading to a "brain-sparing" effect. The brain-sparing effect is a feature of asymmetric growth restriction. However, sometimes the fetus does not get enough nutrition even early in pregnancy. In this case, the fetus may not be able to change her blood vessels to send enough blood flow and nutrition to the brain. In this case, the baby's head and body are both small, which are features of symmetric growth restriction. Genetic syndromes and infections are more likely to cause symmetric growth restriction than asymmetric growth restriction.

Family Story #1: Michelle

My son turned two yesterday, which I'm thankful for because those were some rough times. Happy to be farther and farther away from them.

We first got notice that something was funny at the twenty-week ultrasound. During the ultrasound they said my son's weight was nine ounces. I swore my daughters' weights were much closer to the one-pound mark at the gender-reveal ultrasound. The midwife emailed me two days later and told me that baby had a single umbilical artery (SUA), which I knew nothing about at that point but can now tell you a lot about. She said that since there were no heart issues, it was likely an isolated SUA case, and we'd just do more ultrasounds to check growth. At 26 weeks for the first growth check, they now found that baby had "short long bones." Instead of an email from the midwife, I got a call from my doctor's office for my "high-risk pregnancy" to schedule an in-depth ultrasound. I'm thinking what on earth is going on? I didn't have ANY problems with my first two pregnancies, so this was all new to me.

At the 28-week ultrasound appointment, we learned of the short long bones again, which included the femur and humerus but not the feet and hands necessarily. The SUA was confirmed, and now they also found liver calcifications, which can also occur randomly but are common with infections. At that point I was tested for multiple infections myself (CMV, etc.). At this point, baby was measuring at 55th percentile for overall size, so still pretty normal. Two weeks later at 30 weeks, we found that there were now more problems – placental thickening (also indicative of infection) and a slight cloverleaf head shape. The perinatologist told us that baby likely had one of three things: 1) non-lethal form of dwarfism, 2) growth restriction from placental infection, or 3) some type of chromosomal abnormality that would require follow-up with a geneticist after birth.

That was by far my lowest point. I had no idea why my sweet baby wasn't growing right, and there was absolutely nothing I could do about it. I had postpartum depression and anxiety (PPD/A) with both my daughters but never during pregnancy. This time, I started having bad symptoms of PPD/A from this moment forward. Because so many things were unknown, I honestly didn't know if he'd make it. I didn't know if we were going to be bringing home a baby. I tried to be as excited as I could. We did maternity pictures with my not-very-full belly and had a baby shower with close friends who knew why I wasn't brimming with joy. We set up the Pack 'n Play, but I would cry, as I wondered if he would be with us or if he'd be on oxygen or a feeding tube. Would we be able to send him to day care, or would my husband need to quit his job and stay home with our new son?

Eventually the growth restriction started catching up to him. He dropped from the 55th percentile to the 35th percentile of overall size over the course of a few ultrasounds, which were now an every two weeks kind of thing. At the 36-week ultrasound, I was hoping he wouldn't be under the 10th percent, and he wasn't. They said he was at the 16th percentile. Knowing he'd be small at birth, we had to plan to have him at the hospital across town, the one that had the

NICU, as it was likely he'd need to be resuscitated or spend time at NICU.

At birth, he was 5 pounds 13 ounces, meaning the 8th percentile for being born at 38 weeks 2 days. He was MUCH smaller than my girls, who were 8 pounds 2 ounces at 39 weeks 2 days and 8 pounds 9 ounces at 39 weeks 3 days. He did need some help breathing at birth, but other than that he looked fine, just small. I thought we'd avoided the NICU too since he was breathing and eating, but due to his low blood sugars (25 at around two to three hours after birth and then 19 another hour after that), he had to be taken to NICU for a dextrose intravenous (IV) line.

He stayed in the NICU for ten days. Every time they tried to wean him a little bit, he'd bottom out on his blood sugars again. The doctors didn't want me to try to nurse him because it took too much energy for his poor body, so to the bottle we went. We learned in the NICU that he has hard-to-find veins. His arm IV failed at one point, and they couldn't find any other vein, so they had to use one in his head. That process traumatized him so much that he stopped eating, so he received a nasogastric tube. He was finally able to eat again and wean off the NG tube. Eventually, he weaned off the dextrose IV, too.

They checked my placenta for infections, but there was nothing. They confirmed the SUA and reported a marginal cord insertion – maybe he just got poor blood flow, causing all these problems? At birth the cord was wrapped around his neck twice, and he had a knot (or maybe even two?) within the umbilical cord. They never tested anything else on him related to his genes or the liver calcifications. No X-rays were taken of his bones. So, I still don't know what caused all of this. Or if he had SGA or IUGR. Or if it was related to that pesky SUA? Who knows...?

But he is here, and he is healthy. He crawled and walked later than my girls. He's now two years old and still not talking much, but he tries hard to imitate sounds. He had a very hard time transitioning to solid foods and was found to have a tongue tie, which was revised right before his first birthday. He never had problems nursing or with a bottle, but the solid foods made him choke and gag. Both his height and weight continue to be on the lower end of the spectrum. He's around the third percentile for his weight and somewhere around the eighth to tenth percentile for his height. But he loves puppies. He loves playing with balls of all kinds, playing with his sisters, and singing songs. He never qualified for Early Intervention, even when he was nearly a year old and couldn't feed properly. So, overall, he is a little Rockstar.

Questions and Medical Responses Raised by Michelle's Story

1. Does Miles have growth restriction or is he SGA?

    Miles meets the diagnosis for SGA because his birth weight was less than tenth percentile for his gestational age. In this case, Miles is also likely to have growth restriction because his estimated fetal weight continued to decrease on repeated ultrasound measurements. Persistent and worsening poor growth on ultrasounds is a characteristic of growth restriction. However, most obstetricians do not diagnose a fetus with growth restriction unless the estimated fetal weight falls below the tenth percentile.

2. What are "long bones?"

    Long bones are the bones in the body that are longer than they are wide. The large bones in the arms and legs are long bones. Obstetricians can measure the length of the femur bone, which is located in the thigh, with ultrasound.

3. What are "short long bones?" What is dwarfism?

    "Short long bones" means that the bones of the legs and arms are shorter than expected. Growth restriction is one of the causes of short long bones. Other causes of short long bones are often from changes to the baby's genes. Dwarfism is a condition of short height. Dwarfism can be caused by a variety of genetic and hormonal changes in the baby's body.

4. Why is Miles small?

    As is true in many cases, we may never know why Miles was born small. Michelle mentions that Miles had a single umbilical artery (SUA). Normally there are two umbilical arteries that bring blood from the fetus to the placenta. SUA sometimes is associated with problems with the development of the heart leading to congenital heart disease. However, most often SUA is an isolated finding that does not cause problems with the body's development. Kinks in the umbilical cord may contribute to decreased fetal growth, although how much of an impact this had on Miles is unknown.

5. What is a perinatologist?

    A perinatologist is an obstetrician who specializes in high-risk pregnancies.

6. What is a normal blood sugar level? Why is a normal blood sugar level important? What is dextrose?

    During pregnancy, a fetus gets a continuous infusion of sugar from the placenta. After birth, the constant supply of sugar is stopped, and the baby has to rely on sugar from feeding and the sugar stored in his own body. Small babies do not have as much sugar stored in their bodies and therefore are at higher risk for having a low blood sugar, which is discussed in more detail in Chapter 3. A normal blood sugar for a baby after birth is difficult to define and remains a hotly debated topic among physicians and researchers. However, nearly all nurseries and NICUs will treat a blood sugar less than 40. Low blood sugar levels can cause brain damage, so physicians take blood sugar levels very seriously. Treating a low blood sugar can mean giving the baby a sugar gel and allowing her to continue to eat normally, providing tube feedings of formula or donor mother's milk, providing bottle feeding of formula or donor mother's milk, or providing sugar directly into the vein of the baby with an IV solution. The IV solution is made of dextrose, which is a type of sugar. Donor mother's milk is milk that has been donated by women who are done pumping breastmilk for their own baby. This can happen because the mother produces more milk than her baby needs or because of an infant loss. Donor mother's milk is pasteurized similarly to cow milk in stores. Donor mother's milk also is screened for infections.

7. Should I breastfeed my growth-restricted baby?

Yes, typically a growth-restricted baby can breastfeed successfully. Keeping the baby's blood sugar in a normal range while working on breastfeeding is an art. There is no best way to maintain a baby's blood sugar while working on feedings. If a mother is ok with giving bottles to her baby, and the baby is willing to take a bottle, then bottle feeding is a perfectly acceptable way to feed a baby as well. On the other hand, if the mother prefers to exclusively breastfeed, then that desire should be supported by hospital staff. There are many alternatives to bottle feeding to maintain normal blood sugars, and these alternatives are discussed in more detail in Chapter 3.

8. Is it typical for a growth-restricted baby not to meet development milestones like walking and talking on time?

While most babies who have growth restriction do not have delayed development, growth-restricted babies are at higher risk for not meeting developmental milestones like walking and talking. Development is discussed in greater detail in Chapter 5.

9. What services are available for babies with developmental delays?

All states offer a program called early intervention or something similar to early intervention. Depending on the state, these programs are either free or low-cost to most families. Often these programs will see babies and young children in the home to do an evaluation and provide necessary therapies. However, only babies and children who meet certain criteria for severity of developmental problems will qualify for services. Your pediatrician can guide you to find the most appropriate services in your area.

CHAPTER 2

How Is Growth Restriction Diagnosed and Managed during Pregnancy?

Obstetricians and midwives use a variety of techniques to monitor a fetus's growth. One of these techniques is the fundal height, which is the measurement from the mother's pubic bone to the top of her uterus. The fundal height is measured using a measuring tape on the mother's belly. Between 16- and 36-weeks' gestation, the fundal height in centimeters should be approximately equal to the number of weeks of gestation. For example, the fundal height of a 16-week old fetus should be about 16 cm. If the uterus is smaller than expected, further investigation may be done to determine why the uterus is measuring small. A small uterus may be caused by the small size of the fetus, low amounts of amniotic fluid, which is the fluid surrounding the baby, and inaccurate measurements. We will focus on the small size of the fetus.

When there is a concern that the fetus is small, the next test that obstetrical providers usually perform is an ultrasound.

An ultrasound provides useful information about fetal size and growth and may help obstetricians understand why the fetus is not growing as expected. Obstetricians can measure the fetal head size, circumference around the abdomen, and length of the femur bone in the thigh. They also can estimate the fetal body weight with an ultrasound. Obstetricians plot these measurements on a chart to track how the fetus is growing over time (**Figure 6**).

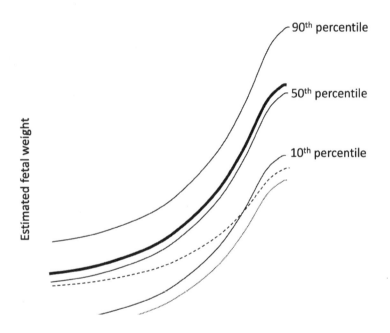

Growth chart during pregnancy. Typical baby growth during pregnancy (thick solid line), a baby with growth restriction (dashed line), and a baby who is small for gestational age (dotted line).

Figure 6

For example, an average fetus with average weight gain may follow along the 60th percentile throughout pregnancy. This means that the fetus is larger than six of every ten fetuses for that gestational age, and smaller than four of every ten fetuses for that gestational age. If the weight of this fetus decreases significantly below the 60th percentile as the baby grows, this can be a concern to obstetricians. Since fetal body weight is an estimate, the measurements can be significantly different than the actual weight when the baby is born, particularly if these estimates are made later in gestation. However, if there is a concern about how well the fetus is growing, obstetricians often perform multiple ultrasounds during pregnancy. Ultrasound measurements are more accurate when more than one ultrasound is done.

Ultrasounds also can be used to measure how blood flows through the umbilical cord and ductus venosus. The ductus venosus is a blood vessel that carries nutrient- and oxygen-rich blood from the umbilical cord to the baby's heart. The umbilical blood flow measurements indicate if the blood is flowing normally from the placenta to the fetus and back again or if the blood stops or even reverses direction between heart beats (**Figure 7**). This stopping or reversal of blood flow is called "absence of end diastolic flow" or "reversal of end diastolic flow." Absence and reversal of end diastolic flow may indicate that the fetus is having problems and may prompt obstetricians to consider delivering the fetus, even if he is not yet full term.

Ultrasound also may show the underlying reason that an infant has growth restriction. Certain genetic syndromes or viruses that cause a fetus to be small can cause changes in the rest of the body. Some of these changes can be seen on ultrasound images and may indicate what is causing growth restriction. For example, changes in how the brain appears on an ultrasound can indicate that the fetus has an infection with cytomegalovirus (CMV). Alternatively, structural changes in the heart on an ultrasound may indicate that the fetus has congenital heart disease. Other tests such as genetic or viral tests can be done on fluid obtained from around the fetus. The fluid from around the fetus is collected through a procedure called an amniocentesis. Some testing for genetic and infectious causes also can be done on the mother's blood.

Checking the mother's blood pressure is important when the fetus has growth restriction. If the mother's blood pressure is high, additional tests may be done on the mother's blood and urine for further evaluation. These tests help to determine if the mother has high blood pressure from causes such as preeclampsia, pregnancy-induced hypertension, or HELLP (Hemolysis, Elevated Liver enzymes, and Low Platelets) syndrome. Pregnancy-induced hypertension is high blood pressure during but not before pregnancy. Preeclampsia is most often diagnosed when a mother has high blood pressure and protein in her urine. HELLP syndrome is a severe form of preeclampsia in which the mother has high blood pressure, abnormal liver tests, and low platelets, which are the parts of the blood that form blood clots.

If the obstetricians and midwives are concerned that the baby has growth restriction, the mother may be sent to a specialist in a field called maternal-fetal medicine. Maternal-fetal medicine specialists, who are also known as perinatologists, specialize in high-risk pregnancies such as ones in which the fetus has growth restriction. Perinatologists

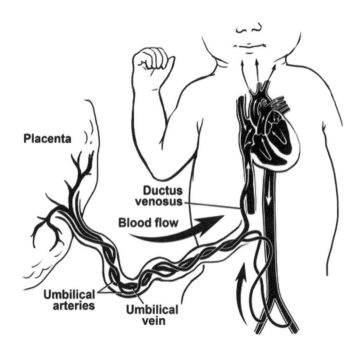

*Blood flows from the placenta to the fetus through the umbilical cord
in the umbilical vein, then to the ductus venosus, and then to the fetus's
heart. Blood flows back to the placenta from the fetus through
the umbilical cord in the umbilical arteries.*

Figure 7

sometimes can help determine what caused the growth
restriction and therefore what the parents can expect in their
baby's future. Often, however, the cause of growth restriction remains unknown. Sometimes the perinatologist is a
consultant for the mother's primary obstetrician, and other
times the perinatologist becomes the primary obstetrician for
the mother's high-risk pregnancy.

The health of a fetus also may be assessed with non-stress tests (NSTs) and biophysical profiles (BPPs). Non-stress tests are tracings of the fetal heart rate. The fetus should have a baseline heart rate in the normal range for gestational age, which is usually between 120 and 160 beats per minute. The fetus's heart rate is typically higher earlier in pregnancy and lower later in pregnancy. Non-stress tests also measure the number of times that the fetal heart rate increases by fifteen beats per minute above the fetus's baseline heart rate for at least ten to fifteen seconds at a time. This increase in heart rate is called an "acceleration." It is normal for a fetus to have at least two episodes of acceleration during the twenty minutes of non-stress testing. If the fetus has less than two accelerations, the test is called "non-reactive." Non-reactive non-stress test results can be normal if the fetus is sleeping, but non-reactive results also can indicate that the fetus is in distress. If the obstetrician is concerned about the results of the non-stress test, a biophysical profile measurement may be performed next.

A BPP is a series of ultrasound measurements that includes the non-stress test information (**Figure 8**). The five tests in a BPP are an NST, breathing movements, body movements, muscle tone, and amniotic fluid levels. Breathing movements, body movements, and muscle tone are measured during a thirty-minute period. Breathing movements measure whether the fetus's lungs expand for at least thirty seconds during the thirty-minute period on ultrasound. Body movements measure whether the fetus's body moves at least three times. Muscle tone measures whether a limb fully extends and returns to a resting position at least once. Amniotic fluid levels are scored as normal if there is at least one pocket of a normal fluid level. A fetus receives either two points for each category with normal findings or zero points for each category with abnormal findings. There is no score of one point for these measurements. Since there are five categories, a fetus can have a score from zero to ten. The way obstetricians manage a pregnancy with an abnormal BPP score often depends on the specific BPP score and the gestational age of the fetus. In general, lower BPP scores are more concerning for the fetus not getting enough oxygen from the placenta. Lower BPP scores are more likely to prompt repeated testing or delivery of the fetus, even if preterm. Your healthcare practitioner will discuss recommendations and options based on your and your baby's individual circumstances.

Category	Normal finding
Reactive heart rate	At least two episodes of acceleration in 30 minutes (NST)
Breathing movements	At least one episode of breathing in 30 minutes
Body movements	At least three movements in 30 minutes
Muscle tone	At least one episode of fully extending a limb and returning to resting position (for example, opening and closing a hand) in 30 minutes
Amniotic fluid levels	At least one pocket of normal fluid levels

*Biophysical profile categories. For each category,
a normal score is 2 points, and an abnormal score is 0 points.*

Figure 8

Your doctor may ask you to keep a log of your baby's activity. Your doctor will instruct you about when to call or seek immediate medical attention if you notice certain changes in how your baby moves. Decreased movement of your baby may be a sign of distress that needs urgent intervention, which may mean urgent delivery even if your baby is premature. Prematurity is defined as delivery before 37 weeks. Your doctor will discuss the options, benefits, and risks with you so that you can make the most informed decision for you and your baby.

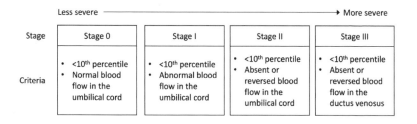

Stages of intrauterine growth restriction.

Figure 9

Growth and ultrasound measurements can be classified into stages of growth restriction (**Figure 9**). Stage 0 growth restriction includes fetuses with a fetal weight or abdominal circumference less than the tenth percentile for gestational age and normal blood flow in the umbilical cord and brain. Many SGA but healthy fetuses fall into this category, but this category also includes some growth-restricted fetuses. Stage I through III growth restriction includes fetuses with a fetal weight or abdominal circumference less than the tenth percentile for gestational age and progressively more severe blood flow findings on ultrasound.

Interventions for growth restriction depend partly on the stage of growth restriction. With worsening degrees of umbilical blood flow, most obstetricians and perinatologists will recommend more frequent NSTs, inpatient intensive monitoring, or early delivery. Your healthcare practitioner will recommend a course of action based on your and your baby's particular health history and circumstances.

Pregnant mothers with Stage I, II, and III growth-restricted fetuses often are given an injection of betamethasone, a steroid that helps to protect the baby's brain after birth and induces the fetal lungs to produce surfactant, which is a soapy substance that helps to keep the baby's lungs open after birth. Betamethasone is given as two injections 24 hours apart into the muscles of the pregnant mother. Timing the first dose of betamethasone can be tricky, as the most beneficial effects of betamethasone on the baby's brain and lungs occur 48 hours to approximately one to two weeks after the first injection. Your doctor will talk to you about the best timing of betamethasone injections, if they are required.

Research studies show that fetuses with Stage 0 or Stage I growth restriction nearly always survive to delivery. Such intensive follow-up and intervention are done in Stage II and Stage III growth-restricted fetuses because up to half of fetuses with Stage III growth restriction will not survive to be born. Fetuses with Stage II growth restriction have better survival than fetuses with Stage III growth restriction but are still at risk of not surviving to be born. Despite these scary numbers, fetuses can survive for weeks with reversal of end diastolic flow in the ductus venosus in Stage III growth restriction. If possible, most obstetricians will try to give both doses of betamethasone before delivering the baby to give the baby the best chance at being healthier after birth. Your doctor will discuss with you the risks and potential benefits of delivering your baby early based on the specific medical information about your pregnancy, results of ultrasounds and other testing, and your wishes for your baby.

There are no consistently, across-the-board effective treatment options for growth restriction, although researchers are still looking. If a mother's health condition is contributing to the growth restriction, obstetricians may work with other specialists to try to improve her health. Mothers with preeclampsia or who are at high risk for preeclampsia are often given low-dose aspirin to improve blood flow to the placenta. Sometimes obstetricians recommend oxygen and bed rest, although there is not good data in the medical literature that either will work well to improve growth restriction. Vitamins and nutrition supplements work only for women who are themselves severely malnourished. Sometimes improved nutrition may prolong pregnancy, but it does not improve or prevent growth restriction. In fact, certain kinds of nutrition supplements may be harmful. Researchers are studying several medications to evaluate whether they may improve or prevent growth restriction, but these medications are still being investigated and are not available yet.

What Parents Can Do

As parents of a baby recently diagnosed with growth restriction, the emotional turmoil of learning that something is possibly wrong with your baby may be made so much harder by not knowing the reason for the growth restriction. Potentially making matters worse, parents, especially mothers, often blame themselves for their baby's condition. Remember that no one wakes up in the morning thinking that they do not want the best for their children, and you are no different. Growth restriction is not your fault. If your lifestyle choices, such as smoking or using illicit drugs, are contributing to your baby's growth restriction, use that information as a motivation to change and to get yourself into a healthier place for both you and your baby.

Parents can educate and inform themselves about what growth restriction means for them. As they get more information about why their baby has growth restriction, parents can learn about the specific causes and prepare themselves for potential upcoming challenges. A baby with growth restriction from pre-eclampsia has different future health challenges compared with one who has trisomy 13. One of these challenges may include delivering before term and having the baby admitted to the NICU. There are great resources to help guide parents through the NICU stay and make that transition less overwhelming (see **Appendix 1** – Resources for Parents).

Lastly, ask questions. It is ok to ask the same question to as many medical providers as you can until you feel that your question is fully answered. You will get slightly different answers from each provider, but that's ok as long as the overall message is the same. As you get more answers, you'll probably feel more comfortable with the upcoming challenges in your and your baby's lives.

Family Story #2: Sandra

Our son was born at 2.1 kg (4 pounds, 10 ounces). His low before we left the hospital was 1.95 kg (4 pounds, 4.8 ounces). He was born at 39 weeks 4 days gestational age. I'm pretty sure of the date since I practiced the Fertility Awareness Method and know when I ovulated and conceived, so our dates weren't off.

My pregnancy was relatively complicated, although not to the degree that I needed extended bedrest. I had two miscarriages before I fell pregnant with Craig, our son. The first was probably due to deworming medication. We live in South Africa, and our dogs live in the house with us. It's not unhygienic, but I have been deworming us on a regular basis since we got the dogs three years prior. I didn't check the insert since I specifically told the pharmacist I'm pregnant and he assured me it was safe. Turns out deworming medication is fetotoxic in rats, so it's probably the reason for the first miscarriage. We saw a normal heartbeat at about seven weeks, but I started bleeding on and off at eight weeks. At ten weeks there was no heartbeat. I had a dilation and curettage (D&C), and we fell pregnant within a month or two. This time, I fear it was an ectopic pregnancy. My beta-hCG wasn't increasing like it should have. I went in for three blood draws in a week and presented the results to my gynecologist. He gave me a shot of methotrexate since I was very reluctant to go for surgery. Of course, I had to wait three months after that to fall pregnant, and in month four, I did fall pregnant. Everything seemed normal, but at eight weeks I had a very strong bleed and went to see the gynecologist that morning. He checked and by that time most of the bleeding had cleared up. From the ultrasound he said that it looked like I had a vanishing twin pregnancy. At twelve weeks, I went for the typical twelve-week scan and associated bloodwork. The gynecologist said from the ultrasound everything looked perfect. A week later, I received a phone call from him because the bloodwork showed that our baby was at an elevated risk for Edwards Syndrome – 1/32 risk. So, we went in for an amniocentesis. The obstetrician was concerned by the color of my amniotic fluid. I remember we went in for the results on my birthday. I was so nervous and scared. It turns out our baby was 100% a boy with no genetic issues. I am an asthmatic but continued to see my pulmonologist more regularly during my pregnancy. He was happy with my lungs throughout the pregnancy. My blood pressure was low, if anything, and there was no indication that anything was amiss up until about 34 weeks' gestational age. Our son had pretty much stopped gaining weight at that stage, although we only realized it at 36 weeks at my next appointment. Our obstetrician was concerned but not overly so. He made me go for a weekly cardiotocography (CTG), which checks the movement and heart rate. I wanted to have a vaginal birth, so we waited. At 38 weeks he wanted me to go in every second day, and at 39 weeks I went in daily. On a Sunday, I saw something was off with our baby's heart rate and movement.

The CTG was showing that he was going into fetal distress. I told the nurse it didn't look right, and she said she'll show the obstetrician. Of course, that Monday I went back, and the same pattern was there. I was getting more concerned. At 8 PM on the Monday evening, the nurse phoned and said the obstetrician wanted me admitted for observation. So, I went in. At 11 PM she had me do another CTG, and at 2 AM on the Tuesday she said to phone your husband because the obstetrician wanted an emergency C-section. I was not about to mess around with induction with a baby that's already distressed, so at 2:32 he was born, 2.1kg (4 pounds, 10 ounces). He was covered in meconium but breathed on his own and started crying as soon as he was born. He was the skinniest baby I had ever seen for a full-term baby. He was so hungry and crying for food all the time. Thankfully I didn't have any issues with milk production once my milk came in, and he nursed like a champ. At three months old he was such a cute chubby baby.

The health issues that we experienced later on were mostly pulmonary. He has a deviated septum, so he always had a postnasal drip, which caused him to be admitted with pneumonia at two years three months. He had a throat infection and I had such trouble getting him to swallow the antibiotics that he never properly finished the course, even though I'm usually obsessive about it. He ended up with bacterial pneumonia. Asthma runs in our family, so I can't really say whether the current lungs issues are related to the genetic predisposition to asthma, his pneumonia at just over two years old, or his low birth weight. I took him to a pediatric pulmonologist when he was four to five years old. His asthma is very well-controlled at the moment. He's such a skinny kid. He's now just over 130cm (four feet, three inches) tall, and weighs 25kg (55 pounds). He's not emaciated by any means, but he's definitely skinnier than most kids his age. He's healthy otherwise. He's doing incredibly well at school and is active. He does hockey, cricket, and karate. He's not as strong or muscular as other kids his age, but he's active and healthy, which is all I can want.

Questions and Medical Responses Raised by Sandra's Story

1. Is Craig SGA? Is he growth restricted?

   Craig was born with a weight less than the tenth percentile for a full-term baby, so Craig is SGA. Craig is also likely to be growth restricted because his growth slowed in the last few weeks of pregnancy.

2. What is CTG?

   Cardiotocography (CTG) is another name for a non-stress test.

3. What is Edwards Syndrome?

   Edwards Syndrome is a genetic condition caused by an extra copy of chromosome 18. Many babies with Edwards Syndrome are growth restricted, and therefore it is one of the causes of growth restriction that physicians look for in a baby with growth restriction.

4.   What is low birth weight?

Low birth weight is a birth weight less than 2500 grams or 5 pounds 8 ounces.

5.   Did Craig's small size at birth contribute to his pneumonia at two years old?

It is possible that Craig's small size at birth contributed to his pneumonia. The immune system in babies with growth restriction often does not work normally, which can lead to an increased chance that these babies may have some difficulty fighting infections in childhood. The type of infections are similar to infections normally found in children, but they can happen more frequently.

6.   Is a deviated septum or asthma associated with growth restriction?

Growth restriction is not associated with a deviated septum. However, growth restriction may be associated with asthma, although there is some conflicting research on this association.

CHAPTER 3

What Are Effects of Growth Restriction in Full-term Newborns?

Most babies born with growth restriction are born at or near term, and most are healthy. This chapter will discuss what medical challenges your baby may face now that she is born and what testing may be done both to determine why your baby developed growth restriction and to help your baby be healthy. The next chapter will discuss more specifics about what happens if your baby is born prematurely and ways in which prematurity has the potential to complicate the medical challenges that can be associated with growth restriction.

Testing to determine why a baby has growth restriction may be done after birth if the reason the baby is small remains unknown. Sometimes if a small baby appears to be healthy, doctors and parents may decide not to pursue any further testing to determine the cause of the growth restriction.

The tests done to determine why your baby had growth restriction depend on whether your baby has any other features of either an infection or a genetic syndrome. If your baby has features that suggest a reason for having growth restriction, then your medical provider will likely order tests specific to these findings. If no specific cause is suggested based on your baby's physical exam, then often a urine or saliva test for cytomegalovirus (CMV) is ordered. CMV is tested for because it can cause progressive hearing loss and treatment is available to limit the progression of hearing loss caused by CMV. Testing also may be done on the placenta after birth. A pathologist, which is a specialist in examining body tissues, can examine the placenta visually and under a microscope. Sometimes examination of the placenta reveals a cause for growth restriction, such as a small placenta or a placenta with a blood clot that limits oxygen and nutrition delivery to the fetus. Despite testing for these and other conditions, a reason for why a baby has growth restriction is not always found.

Babies with growth restriction are more likely to have certain medical challenges soon after birth. These challenges may include hypoglycemia (low blood sugar), hypothermia (low body temperature), polycythemia (high red blood cell counts), jaundice (yellow coloring of the skin), and asphyxia (decreased oxygen and increased acid levels in the blood). The most common medical challenges that full-term babies with growth restriction face are low blood sugar and jaundice.

Low blood sugar occurs more commonly in newborns with growth restriction than in newborns without growth restriction. During a typical pregnancy, babies slowly build up sugar stores in their liver. After birth, while waiting for her mother's milk to come in and learning how to eat, the baby uses these stores of sugar in the liver to maintain a normal blood sugar level. A normal blood sugar level ensures normal delivery of sugar to important organs like the heart and brain. Because of the robust stores of sugar in the liver, most babies transition from being in the womb to eating mother's milk without any complications. Growth-restricted babies can be different. Growth-restricted babies tend to have less sugar stored in the liver because instead of storing sugar in the liver, they use the sugar that they received through the placenta to grow as best they can. Because growth-restricted babies may have less sugar stored in the liver, they are more likely to have a low blood sugar after birth. This low blood sugar level may require intervention to help maintain a normal blood sugar level. A low blood sugar level may lead to brain damage, so physicians take blood sugar levels seriously.

Different hospitals may have different ways to manage low blood sugar, but the overall goal is to provide the baby with enough sugar to maintain a normal blood sugar level while she learns how to eat. Interventions may include giving a sugar-containing gel solution to the baby by mouth, which should be followed by a feeding of mother's milk or formula; providing formula or donated human milk to the baby by bottle or by temporary feeding tube after breastfeeding; using a supplemental nursing system (SNS) including a tube with formula or donated milk placed into the baby's mouth during breastfeeding; or by placing an IV line and giving sugar directly into the baby's veins. All of these methods are effective in treating low blood sugar, but the gel solution or supplemental tube feeding may need to be repeated to keep your baby's blood sugar in the normal range. Depending on the hospital where you baby was born, sometimes placing an IV or a feeding tube will require admission to the NICU. The good news is that once a baby starts to eat well, the blood sugar usually normalizes without the need for further intervention. In a few cases, babies need to have extra calories mixed in with the feedings for a few weeks or months to keep their blood sugar in the normal range. The extra calories are added into a bottle or tube feeding by mixing either mother's milk or formula with either a powder or a liquid fortifier. The fortifier adds extra calories and minerals to the mother's milk or formula and is somewhat similar to an adult drinking a protein shake. The fortified feeding is then given to the baby with a bottle or using a SNS at home. Signs that your baby may have a low blood sugar include jitteriness or shakiness, excessive sleepiness or difficulty in getting your baby to wake up for feedings, low muscle tone or floppy muscles, and a lack of interest in feeding. If you notice any of these symptoms, notify your medical provider right away.

Growth-restricted babies also have less subcutaneous fat, which is fat under the skin, than babies without growth restriction. Having enough subcutaneous fat is what makes babies have a classic chubby baby appearance. Subcutaneous fat helps insulate our bodies and keep us warm. Growth-restricted babies are therefore more likely to have challenges keeping their body temperature in the normal range. The calories that babies eat are used primarily for three things: first, to maintain a normal body temperature; second, to maintain a normal blood sugar; and third, to grow. Babies with less subcutaneous fat use more calories to stay warm and maintain a normal body temperature. If the baby uses more of her calories for warmth instead of growth, the baby often won't grow as well. If a growth-restricted baby is not growing well after birth, sometimes physicians will warm up the baby either with a warmer or an incubator. Once the baby can grow and gain more subcutaneous fat, the baby will be able to maintain her own body temperature without extra help from these devices. One of the requirements for discharge from the hospital for a baby who has required a device to keep warm is that she must maintain her body temperature and gain weight without supplemental heat.

Babies with growth restriction are also at a higher risk for needing oxygen after birth because they often have thicker blood due to extra red blood cells. New red blood cells, which are the oxygen-carrying and oxygen-delivering cells of the body, are made in the bone marrow. The bone marrow is the fatty middle part of bones in the body. Production of new red blood cells in the bone marrow depends on the amount of oxygen in the body. When oxygen levels in the fetus are low, which is common in growth restriction, the kidneys are stimulated to produce a compound called erythropoietin. Erythropoietin stimulates the bone marrow to make more red blood cells. The extra red blood cells may be beneficial to the growth-restricted fetus because the fetus will likely get more oxygen from the placenta through the greater number of oxygen-carrying red blood cells. However, high levels of red blood cells also can increase the blood's viscosity, which is its thickness. A higher viscosity of blood makes it harder to get oxygen into the body after birth because the high number of red blood cells have difficulty squeezing through the small blood vessels in the lungs. For this reason, growth-restricted babies with high numbers of red blood cells are more likely to need oxygen after birth. Physicians measure the number of red blood cells with a blood test called a hematocrit. Generally, a hematocrit level higher than 70–75% if the baby is on room air or 65–70% if the baby is on oxygen is considered to be too high. A high hematocrit can be treated by a procedure called a partial exchange transfusion. A partial exchange transfusion removes a small amount of the baby's blood and extra red blood cells and replaces the blood with saline, an IV fluid that contains salt and water. A partial exchange transfusion is overall a safe procedure, although a partial exchange transfusion requires an IV to be placed. Red blood cells use blood sugar for survival. In addition to the reasons for low blood sugar discussed earlier in this chapter, a high number of red blood cells can increase the risk of low blood sugar after birth.

Many healthy full-term newborns may develop jaundice. Jaundice is the yellow color that skin temporarily develops a few days after birth and typically lasts until about two weeks of life. Most of the time jaundice goes away on its own and does not need treatment. Bilirubin is the compound that causes jaundice. Bilirubin is produced by the normal process of red blood cells breaking down after birth. Growth-restricted babies are more likely to have high bilirubin levels because they are more likely to have high numbers of red blood cells. After birth, the extra red blood cells are broken down in the body and release higher amounts of bilirubin into the blood. Physicians measure bilirubin levels to evaluate whether the bilirubin level needs to be treated. High levels of bilirubin can cause hearing loss and a type of brain damage called kernicterus, so physicians take high bilirubin levels seriously. Symptoms of high bilirubin include low muscle tone (floppy), decreased interest in eating, a high-pitched cry, and in more severe cases, muscle stiffening, arching of the back, and seizures.

Treatment for high bilirubin levels is usually quite easy and is done with special lights in a process called phototherapy. The blue wavelength in the light changes bilirubin into a form that can be excreted in the urine. This makes it easier for the baby's body to eliminate the excess bilirubin. Historically, physicians would recommend exposing the baby to sunlight or placing the baby's crib near a window to decrease the bilirubin levels, but this practice is no longer recommended because of the potential for ultraviolet light damage or sunburn to a baby's sensitive skin. If bilirubin levels are very high or are not responding quickly to phototherapy, a more intensive process called a double volume exchange transfusion can be done. A double volume exchange transfusion is the process of removing a small amount of the baby's blood and replacing it with the same volume of donated blood. Fortunately, with the technological advancements made in phototherapy lights and physicians' awareness of the severe consequences of high bilirubin levels, the need for a double volume exchange transfusion, as well as the incidence of the more serious effects of high bilirubin, like kernicterus, have dramatically decreased over the past several decades.

Some babies with growth restriction may require delivery by cesarean section due to low levels of oxygen. Most fetuses with growth restriction have decreased levels of oxygen in their blood. Contractions of the uterus during labor can decrease the oxygen delivered to the fetus further.

Because of the decreased oxygen delivered to the fetus during labor, obstetricians will monitor growth-restricted babies specifically for their ability to tolerate labor. Fortunately, many growth-restricted fetuses can tolerate labor and be born vaginally. But if the obstetrician finds evidence that the baby is not tolerating labor, he or she will likely recommend a cesarean section. In rare cases, the additional stress of the fetus not getting enough oxygen during labor combined with chronically low levels of oxygen in growth-restricted fetuses can result in asphyxia. Asphyxia is a severe decrease in oxygen. If it is left untreated, it can lead to coma or death. Asphyxia can lead to impairment of many organs in the body, including the heart, blood vessels, kidneys, lungs, liver, and brain. Most of the body's organs can recover from asphyxia with enough medical support. Many babies with asphyxia from labor and birth can wean off of the extra medical support within one to two weeks of life. However, in severe cases, a baby's body may be too injured to recover despite receiving medical support.

Unfortunately, the damage done to the brain from asphyxia is not always fully reversible. In addition to the injury done directly to the brain from asphyxia, there can be other effects of asphyxia such as swelling and inflammation. If your baby's doctor is concerned that your baby may have asphyxia, then treatment to help the brain may be done. The only treatment currently available to help the baby's brain after asphyxia is called therapeutic hypothermia, or "cooling." Therapeutic hypothermia is a process of cooling a baby's body temperature down to about 92°F for three days. This process allows the brain to rest and heal. Research has shown that because cooler temperatures can help the brain rest and heal, babies who are cooled after asphyxia have better development than babies who are not.

What Parents Can Do

The most important thing for new parents to do is to enjoy your new baby! Congratulations! Most likely your tiny but mighty baby will do well, and you will take home a healthy bundle of joy.

Breastfeeding or bottle-feeding expressed breast milk, if that is the mother's preference, is highly encouraged for growth-restricted infants. Breastfeeding can support long-term development for all babies, including babies with growth restriction. Even if extra calories need to be given to your small baby either to improve growth or to maintain a normal blood sugar level, you can give your baby bottles of breastmilk fortified with extra calories, and your baby still will get all of the benefits of breastmilk. Most hospitals have lactation specialists, who will meet with mothers to help establish breastfeeding or help with pumping breast milk and mixing in extra calories.

If your baby has signs of a low blood sugar, such as jitteriness, sleepiness, or not eating well, ask your provider if checking a blood sugar is appropriate. If your baby has low blood sugar, ask your providers what options are available for providing sugar to your baby, such as bottle feeding, tube feeding, sugar gel, or IV sugar. If you are working on establishing breastfeeding, you may not want to give your baby a bottle. However, understand that in certain hospitals, placing a feeding tube or an IV may require admission to the NICU, which means that your baby will not be in the room with you to work on breastfeeding. You can certainly work on breastfeeding in the NICU, though typically the environment is not as private, calm, or quiet as your room. Do not be afraid to change the plan or to ask your provider to change the plan for how you are going to treat your baby's low blood sugar. For example, if you decide to give a bottle after breastfeeding, but your baby isn't eating well, then the bottle feeding will not help your baby maintain a normal blood sugar.

Another important thing for parents to do after the birth of your growth-restricted baby is to be an advocate for your child. If you see any of the signs of low blood sugar or high bilirubin mentioned in this chapter, let your medical provider know right away. If you do not feel that you are getting the response that you need, let your medical provider know what your worry is and why you feel that it is important to investigate. Sometimes in these cases, even minutes can make a difference in a baby's long-term development, so it is important to voice your concerns.

Family Story #3: Catie

My first pregnancy seemed to be normal. The anatomy scan at 20 weeks was on track. No growth problems were detected. I went into labor at 38.5 weeks, and my son surprised everyone by being born at only 5 pounds 1 ounce. He was labeled "SGA" or "small for gestational age." Not knowing anything was wrong, I delivered at my regional hospital, so he had to be life-flighted to a level 4 NICU in a bigger city due to life-threatening low blood sugar that wouldn't rise with a glucose IV. It was absolutely terrifying to send my two-day old baby on a helicopter without me. I remember being in complete shock. There were so many unknowns, and I was separated from my baby. By the time we got to the NICU and spent the day getting him checked in and evaluated by the neonatologists, I hadn't slept in almost three days after a very long labor. We stayed ten days in the NICU. Those days are a complete blur of sleep deprivation, shock of having a long hospital stay when we hadn't planned for one, and emotions gone haywire from postpartum hormones and the stress of not getting to hold our baby at home like we had planned. Pumping was a challenge I was completely unprepared to face. However, his sugars bounced right up, he gained weight quickly, and he's doing great now as a happy two-and-a-half-year-old! He thankfully didn't have any growth problems at all after birth and has been growing on a regular growth chart just fine since.

Due to my history, for my second pregnancy I was referred to a maternal fetal medicine (MFM) specialist by my obstetrician. My obstetrician told me that it most likely wouldn't happen again but that the MFM would provide extra monitoring at the beginning and once again at the end, just to be safe. At nine weeks, baby measured at the correct size according to my last menstrual period (LMP). At fourteen weeks, baby was already less than five percent and continued to fall from there. We received our official IUGR diagnosis. At 24 weeks, ultrasound detected abnormal umbilical cord flow resistance, I started weekly fetal surveillance with a non-stress tests, plus a biophysical profile ultrasound, which later was upped to twice weekly. My MFM is an hour and a half drive away from my hometown. The appointments took two full hours, so twice weekly surveillance appointments basically became my new part-time job. I was told to be packed and ready to deliver at any appointment if baby showed any signs of distress. It was completely terrifying. Although it was extremely stressful to constantly be fearing for my baby's life, I also felt a deep peace knowing that we were receiving excellent care and that my doctor was doing everything possible to be sure we timed delivery at the most successful point, while not risking keeping her in too long. I was told to do hourly kick counts while awake and to notify the doctor if she seemed to slow down in movement at all.

We pressed on to 33 weeks, but baby was less than one percent and not growing much. She was so tiny that my doctor really wanted to get me to 35 weeks to up her chances of survival. I was given steroids and hospitalized for twice-daily non-stress tests and a once-daily biophysical profile ultrasound with cord flow dopplers. My stay at the hospital was full of anxiety, but I knew I was right where I needed to be. At 35 weeks exactly, they decided it was too risky to keep her in after my fluid levels started to drop and her non-stress tests passed but were less reactive. I delivered her that day. She was 3 pounds 5 ounces, which was so tiny for her gestational age. She only needed a CPAP for a few days and then an oxygen cannula for a few days after, which was such a relief! She had to have a PICC line for IV nutrition, which really scared us, but it was what was best for her. When she was about a week old and had gained a bit of weight from the IV nutrition, we were able to start fortified breastmilk by NG tube and eventually by bottle. Pumping and learning to nurse in the NICU was definitely much easier the second time around, so I had a great supply built up for her. She spent three weeks in the NICU, mostly just to grow and learn to feed.

She proved to us that she really just needed to be born and was not getting the nutrition she needed inside. She doubled her birth weight by seven weeks old and tripled her birth weight by fifteen weeks old. By the time she was nine months old, our pediatrician had her on a regular growth chart, not even one adjusted for gestational age, and she was at the 25th percentile. She has been a bit speech delayed, but otherwise she hit all of her milestones and even walked before the age my son did!

After her pregnancy, because I had two IUGR pregnancies, my obstetrician suggested I be tested for autoimmune disorders. I unfortunately tested positive for lupus and antiphospholipid antibody syndrome (APS), which is a blood-clotting disorder that causes a host of pregnancy complications, including pregnancy loss and IUGR. I got in with a rheumatologist who specializes in pregnancy complications. She started me on lupus medications and recommended blood thinner injections if we had another to prevent IUGR and pregnancy loss. A year later when we were ready for another, we did preconception counseling with my MFM, and he agreed.

We started our third pregnancy with high hopes. Having a diagnosis and treatment plan in place surely meant it would be better this time? They were watching me very closely, and baby measured exactly to my last menstrual period (LMP) at seven weeks and again at ten weeks. At thirteen weeks she started lagging a bit, but they weren't too worried. However, at sixteen weeks baby was only measuring fourteen weeks in size and was at less than one percent. We were not given a great prognosis. They recommended that I up the blood thinner injections to twice daily at the therapy level. At eighteen weeks, I went into preterm labor and found out at the hospital that she had passed away. I had felt her kicking the night before. After birth she was developmentally eighteen weeks, but she still only measured fourteen weeks and a few days, so she had hardly grown at all from her ultrasound done two weeks before. We were completely devastated. Her loss has changed me in ways that I never thought possible. In my research after her birth, I read that antiphospholipid antibody syndrome is one of the main causes of miscarriage and still-birth. I was hoping we could get our rainbow someday. But with this diagnosis and my history, our chances were slim. If we were lucky enough to not lose the baby, there was a great chance that the baby would suffer from IUGR again and would need to be born premature to survive, which comes with a whole other set of complications if it is very early.

For our next pregnancy, I looked into a clinical trial to study an investigational treatment to help prevent growth restriction in women with APS. Unfortunately, I didn't fully meet the lab criteria to be able to participate. My lupus anticoagulant (LA) labs were intermittently positive, so I didn't qualify. But both the trial investigator and my rheumatologist believe that I have APS with positive LA labs and that this trial would benefit me. My rheumatologist was able to procure samples of the drug from the company to allow me to take the drug. It was a LONG pregnancy because the investigational drug had some rough side effects, but we had our first non-IUGR baby back in July!! Our son was 5 pounds 15 ounces at 37 weeks when I was induced. He had no complications, and no NICU stay was needed! It was wonderful. We do believe it's possible that IUGR started right at the very end. I had a growth scan at my MFM three weeks before induction, and he was measuring five and a half pounds. I know the scans can be off, but they were quite careful in measuring multiple times with my history of IUGR. We were expecting him to be at least six and a half pounds. We went back and forth on delivering at 37 or 38 weeks and ultimately decided 37 weeks was best. We were glad that we did. Even though he was still small compared to most babies, he seemed HUGE to us after having such tiny babies before him!

Questions and Medical Responses Raised by Catie's Story

1. What is a growth scan?

   Both growth scans and anatomy scans are ultrasounds that evaluate how well a fetus is doing. Sometimes these terms are used interchangeably, but the purpose of each ultrasound is a little bit different. A growth scan is an ultrasound that evaluates for how well a fetus is growing. An anatomy scan is a fetal ultrasound that is performed specifically to evaluate for fetal development. The purpose of the anatomy scan is to identify potential abnormalities with how the fetus has developed. For example, gastroschisis and congenital heart disease often can be identified with an anatomy scan.

2. What is a neonatologist?

A neonatologist is a physician who specializes in caring for premature and sick newborns. Neonatologists have completed pediatric residency, just like general pediatricians, but then also complete a fellowship in neonatology to learn the specialized care of premature and sick newborns. Neonatologists often only see patients in the NICU, although a few will see mothers in clinics for prenatal counseling of high-risk pregnancies or will see children in the doctor's office who were previously in the NICU.

3. What is CPAP? What is an oxygen cannula?

CPAP stands for continuous positive airway pressure. CPAP is used to help keep a baby's lungs open if a baby is having a difficult time breathing. CPAP is usually given through a tube that sits at the entrance to the baby's nose and connects to a device that provides oxygen and pressure. An oxygen cannula, which is also known as a nasal cannula, looks similar but is usually smaller than CPAP. A nasal cannula does not provide pressure to the lungs but does provide oxygen.

4. What is a PICC line, and why is it used?

PICC line stands for a peripherally inserted central catheter. A PICC line looks similar to a regular IV line on the outside of the body because a PICC line is inserted into one of the veins that a regular IV is inserted into. However, a PICC line is much longer than an IV. A regular IV line is only about one to one-and-a half inches long. A PICC line can be about ten to fifteen inches long. The tip of a PICC line is ideally placed in the large vessels of the body near the heart. These large vessels have more blood flow, which allows physicians to give higher concentrations of sugar through the PICC line than through a regular IV. The higher concentration of sugar is sometimes necessary for babies with a low blood sugar level. PICC lines have other advantages, too. PICC lines last longer than regular IV lines, meaning that the baby will usually not need to be poked as much to get IV access. However, PICC lines also have more risks than a regular IV. Your baby's doctor will talk with you if he or she thinks that a PICC line is necessary for your baby.

5. What is an NG tube?

An NG, or nasogastric, tube is a tube that goes from the baby's nose to her stomach. This type of tube is used to provide feedings of mother's milk or formula to a baby if the baby is not able to eat by mouth. Sometimes babies are not able to eat by mouth because they are too premature to have the skills of eating without inhaling their milk. Other times, the baby may be able to eat by mouth but does not have the stamina to eat orally.

6. What is a level 4 NICU?

NICUs are assigned levels from 1 to 4 according to the level of care provided at each NICU. A level 1 NICU is a well-baby nursery that can take care of healthy newborns. A level 2 NICU can take care of babies who require help breathing, IV fluids, IV medications, and gavage feedings. Level 2 NICUs usually can take care of babies as young as 34 weeks' gestation. A level 3 NICU can take care of all premature babies, often as low as 22 weeks' gestation. Level 3 NICUs also take care of sick babies that require ventilator support and medications to keep blood pressure in the normal range. A level 4 NICU is the most highly specialized NICU. Level 4 NICUs treat babies with the most complex conditions. These conditions often require multiple pediatric subspecialists or surgeons.

7. How often does IUGR happen in subsequent pregnancies?

The risk of having a second baby with growth restriction depends on the mother's health and on why the first baby had growth restriction. For example, if a first baby had growth restriction because the mother smoked during pregnancy, but the mother quit smoking before her second pregnancy, then the likelihood that the second baby will have growth restriction is not as high as if the mother continued to smoke. However, if a first baby had growth restriction because of a health condition such as APS, then the likelihood of a second baby having growth restriction is high. On the other hand, if the first baby had growth restriction because of a congenital heart condition, then the second baby is likely to have growth restriction only if she has a similar congenital heart condition.

CHAPTER 4

What Are Effects of Growth Restriction in Premature Newborns?

Growth-restricted babies are more likely to be delivered prematurely than babies who are not growth restricted. Prematurity is defined as birth before 37 weeks. Early delivery sometimes occurs to help the mother's condition, such as severe preeclampsia. If a mother has preeclampsia, particularly if it is severe, she is more likely to have seizures or convulsions. The only cure for preeclampsia is delivery of the baby. Early delivery also may occur if the baby's health is at risk.

While growth-restricted babies who are born prematurely share the same potential health risks as growth-restricted babies born at full term, premature babies have additional potential health risks that full-term babies do not. The earlier the baby is born, the greater the potential health risks. Most premature babies are born in the late-preterm period, which is between 34- and 36-weeks' gestation. Babies born between 34- and 36-weeks' gestation are at greater risk for developmental problems than babies born at full term, though a family with a term baby and late-preterm baby may not notice the difference between their preterm and term babies. The lungs of babies born between 34 and 36 weeks are not fully mature. These babies may need some oxygen or pressure with CPAP or a breathing machine called a ventilator to keep their lungs open. Depending on the hospital where you deliver your baby, your baby may need to go to the NICU for oxygen treatment. Sometimes babies born in the late-preterm period have difficulty eating and may need IV nutrition or a temporary NG feeding tube from the nose into the stomach to supplement feedings. The good news is that even babies born in the late-preterm period with growth restriction generally do very well.

Babies born at younger ages have more health risks. Babies born at 23- to 24-weeks' gestation, or even at 22-weeks' gestation at some hospitals, are on the other end of prematurity from babies born in the late-preterm period. These babies frequently need to have a breathing tube placed into the lungs, a breathing machine called a ventilator, and medication called surfactant to help the lungs get oxygen into the body. These babies need IV lines, often placed in the blood vessels in the umbilical cord, to give them better nutrition, draw blood for laboratory work, and monitor blood pressure. These babies sometimes need medications to keep their blood pressure normal because they are more likely to have low blood pressure. The blood vessels in the premature brain are leaky and prone to bleeding. Minor bleeding into the brain slightly increases the risk of learning difficulties, but major bleeding into the brain can be devastating for the baby.

Your doctor will monitor a very premature baby for bleeding into the brain with an ultrasound over the fontanelle, which is the soft spot on the top of your baby's head, and discuss the findings with you. This type of ultrasound is usually done around one week of life, but the timing will vary depending on the hospital and on the specific condition of your baby.

Growth restriction can add additional complications for babies born at these very early gestational ages. While premature babies are small, premature babies who have growth restriction are even smaller. Technically, putting in a breathing tube or placing IV lines becomes more challenging for physicians; and if the baby is too small, putting a breathing tube or an IV line in a baby is not possible. There is not an exact cut-off at which a physician is unable to place a breathing tube and IV lines. While you may read stories online of babies who survived when they were born at around 350 grams (three quarters of a pound), most babies who are born this small do not survive because of the difficulty in performing the necessary life-saving measures.

Growth-restricted premature babies are also at greater risk for other conditions unique to premature infants. These conditions include necrotizing enterocolitis (NEC), retinopathy of prematurity (ROP), and chronic lung disease of prematurity (CLD). While premature infants in general are at risk for these conditions, the more premature the baby is born the greater the risk. Growth restriction increases the chance that premature babies will develop these conditions.

NEC is an infection of the intestines that can affect premature newborns. The symptoms of NEC can include bloody stools, intolerance of feedings, a distended abdomen, or green vomit. NEC is treated with IV antibiotics and bowel rest by not feeding the baby and providing nutrition through an IV line. Physicians usually will monitor X-rays of the abdomen about every six hours until NEC is not visible on the X-rays any longer. Usually the bowel is rested and antibiotics are given for seven to ten days. During treatment, your baby may be particularly fussy because he is hungry, which is hard on parents, but most babies tolerate bowel rest quite well. When feedings are started again, usually they will be given in small amounts and slowly increased back to the goal feeding volume. Occasionally surgery is needed to remove a portion of bowel that is severely injured or dead because of the infection that caused NEC. If a significant portion of the bowel died and needs to be removed, the baby may require IV nutrition long-term. In the most severe cases, some babies do not survive the infection despite optimal treatment.

Retinopathy of prematurity is a condition unique to developing eyes. The blood vessels in the back of the eye are sensitive to oxygen levels. Oxygen levels increase after a baby is born, whether the baby is born preterm or full-term. If the blood vessel development is not complete by the time the baby is born, the baby is at risk for abnormal blood vessel development in the eye due to the increased oxygen levels after birth. Most pediatric ophthalmologists, physicians who specialize in children's eyes, begin to examine babies for abnormal blood vessels in the eyes around 32-weeks' corrected gestation. A pediatric ophthalmologist will examine your baby's eyes usually every one to two weeks until the blood vessel development is mature. Occasionally, a baby will need to have surgical intervention for retinopathy of prematurity to prevent blindness. Currently the most common surgical intervention is with laser therapy, but other therapies that are becoming more widely accepted include an injection into the eye with a medication to prevent or correct abnormal blood vessel development.

The term "corrected gestational age" is used two ways. First, the term is used is to put the preterm infant's age into perspective by adding the days after birth to the gestational age at birth. For example, if an infant was born at 28 weeks' gestation and is now three weeks old, then the neonatologist will often say that the infant is 31 weeks corrected gestational age. This correction helps to define milestones for the preterm infant in a more meaningful way. "Corrected gestational age" also can mean that the gestational age is "corrected" for prematurity. For example, if a six-month-old infant was born two months premature, then the infant is only four months corrected gestational age. The prematurity is corrected for by subtracting the infant's degree of prematurity from the current age. This correction is useful when looking at development. A six-month-old infant who was born two months premature should be at the developmental stage of a four-month-old infant, not a six-month-old infant.

Chronic lung disease of prematurity, also known as bronchopulmonary dysplasia (BPD), is a condition in which the lungs have been injured due to prematurity and due to the interventions that neonatologists need to do to keep the baby alive. Necessary interventions – such as oxygen, CPAP, or ventilation – unfortunately induce injury to the developing lung. A baby is diagnosed with chronic lung disease of prematurity if he requires oxygen for the first 28 days of life or if he still requires oxygen at 36-weeks' corrected gestation. While most babies who are diagnosed with chronic lung disease of prematurity wean off of oxygen and go on to live full and healthy lives, some babies have such severe lung disease that they require long-term ventilators to help them breathe. A surgically placed tube through the neck to the lungs, called a tracheostomy, is often placed in these babies to provide the respiratory support the baby needs while still allowing the baby to have optimal development.

What Parents Can Do

Having a baby in the NICU can feel like a roller-coaster. Most babies have good days followed by bad days, and most parents feel like they have little control. There are many NICU-specific resources for families to help you handle the challenges of having a baby in the NICU. Some of these resources are listed at the end of this book. If your small baby requires admission to the NICU, I encourage you to access some of these resources and to connect with other NICU parents if you feel that would be helpful. Remember, most babies who are admitted to the NICU ultimately go on to live full, healthy, and happy lives.

It is entirely possible to successfully breastfeed a premature baby when the premature baby is ready to eat orally. A mother who has a premature baby makes breast-milk that is different from breastmilk that she would make if she had a baby at full term. Premature breastmilk has more protein, among other factors, that help premature babies grow. However, despite the mother's body's attempt to enhance the breastmilk, most premature babies will need to have more calories, protein, and minerals than what preterm breastmilk can provide. Therefore, most NICUs will feed the mother's milk mixed with fortifiers to enhance the calorie, protein, and mineral content of the milk.

Another option for providing extra nutrition at home is to use a transitional formula. Transitional formulas are a special category of formulas that are used usually for premature babies who are ready to go home or for babies who need extra calories. They typically have more calories than regular formulas. Most transitional formulas are sold ready to feed at 22 kilocalories per ounce of formula; whereas, formulas for full-term newborns are sold ready to feed at 19 or 20 kilocalories per ounce. Transitional formulas also have extra minerals compared to full-term formulas. Your doctor may give you instructions on how to mix powdered transitional formula with water to obtain higher calorie concentrations if needed.

Family Story #4: Colby

It was week thirteen of our pregnancy when I received a phone call to discuss the bloodwork results from our first trimester screen. We found out that my PAPP-A levels were very low indicating that my placenta might not be developing correctly. They told me that we would be making an appointment to come back to check the growth of the baby. After scouring the internet for exactly what this might mean for my pregnancy, I found out that having a low PAPP-A level increased our odds of having a baby that was Intrauterine

Growth Restricted (IUGR), as well as a slew of other pregnancy complications such as preeclampsia, placental abruption, and stillbirth. I also learned that this did not definitively mean the baby would be growth restricted since having a low PAPP-A value was not predictive of IUGR, and there are plenty of women who go on to have completely uneventful pregnancies. However, given that my PAPP-A levels were so low, I knew that this did increase my chances.

Every three to four weeks we would go to our MFM doctor for a growth scan of the baby; and although the long bones were measuring shorter than expected, it wasn't until week 26 that our baby boy dropped below the third percentile in size. We immediately knew that something was off because the environment in the room dramatically shifted as the doctor went on to explain to us the severity of the situation we were in. We were to continue growth scans every other week and begin weekly monitoring of the baby through fetal ultrasounds looking at his breathing, movements, heart rate, muscle tone, organs, and the amount of amniotic fluid. We were completely devastated as our worst nightmare had come true. Our baby was severely growth restricted, and all we could do was wait and see what was to come. We started doing a ton of research and found that baby aspirin as well as a high-protein diet were recommended, so we immediately started both after discussing this with our doctor. I had to know that I was doing everything I could possibly do to help my baby's chances of surviving, even though it didn't seem like enough. We knew at this point that we would not make it to full term, and I would have to constantly monitor my baby's movements and come in at the first sign of a decrease since stillbirth was a possibility. We fell into an emotional pattern of hoping for the best while preparing for the worst by buying a couple of preemie outfits and packing our hospital bags to bring to our weekly appointments.

The following growth scan at 28 weeks gave us hope. Our baby's growth was staying in the second percentile, which meant, without any surprises, we would make it to 30 weeks and my baby shower. My husband and I talked about how we never realized how anxious we were at each weekly appointment until we got to hear our baby's heartbeat, and then relief would wash over us. It was as if a giant weight had been lifted off of us only to return a short time after leaving the office. At 29 weeks the doctor discussed with us how the baby's right kidney was enlarged and had been fluctuating between normal and the upper limits of normal for some time but was just something we would continue to monitor along with everything else. He also discussed that as long as this upcoming growth scan looked ok, once we hit the third trimester, we would have to move our growth scans back to every three weeks while still continuing our normal weekly monitoring since the margin of error increases at this stage. He didn't want the baby to appear as if he wasn't growing when he really was. Our 30-week growth scan ended up being a very happy one as our baby made it into the third percentile. The doctor said that making it to 32 weeks is a great milestone since the risk of complications and developmental delays drops dramatically. He also said that week 33 is a critical period of growth for the baby during which my placenta really needs to step up, and if it doesn't, things can change very quickly. Because of this critical period, we were to start coming in twice a week for full biophysical profiles (BPP) and the fetal ultrasound test we normally had but now paired with a non-stress test (NST), which is a test that monitors the fetal heart rate over an extended period of time.

At 33 weeks, we had our growth scan and first NST. My husband and I both felt as though something was off while getting the measurements during our growth scan. Once we finished our NST, the doctor grimly took us back into the ultrasound room to tell us that the baby had dropped below the first percentile. My blood pressure was high, and the NST showed that the baby's heart rate kept dropping. He told us to go to the hospital for further monitoring, and before leaving I was to have my first round of steroid shots administered there in the office to help develop and prep the baby's lungs for delivery, just in case. It is extremely hard to describe the emotional state we were in as we made our way to the hospital. Although we couldn't believe that we might be on our way to deliver our baby, we had been trying to prepare ourselves for this moment for a while now. Being at the hospital felt so surreal, probably because it was all happening so quickly that I couldn't process what was happening fast enough. Once I was hooked up to the fetal monitor, they instantly saw that I was having contractions and that the baby's heart rate dropped in response. Because of these dips in the baby's heart rate, I was admitted for overnight monitoring and the decision on what to do was delayed to the following morning once my MFM doctor came by to do another BPP. That night, no matter what I tried, I couldn't sleep because I was so worried. I couldn't keep myself from constantly listening to my baby's heartbeat, and my contractions were becoming stronger. A couple of times throughout the night the nurse came in to ask me to switch the side that I was lying on, which I later found out is an intervention to try to deliver more oxygen and improve the baby's heart rate. Surprisingly, after that extremely stressful and exhausting night, our doctor told us that the baby's heart rate had improved that morning and he had passed the BPP. We were so shocked and in disbelief that we were actually going to get to go home. Our MFM Doctor said to come back later that day to receive the second round of steroid shots and at this point, if anything else seems off or goes wrong, we will pull the trigger. The OB doctor told me to go home and take off work for the rest for the week but to call anytime if anything remotely felt weird or off. He told me that sometimes mother's intuition is best. From the emotional roller coaster we were on to the minimal sleep the night before, I was so exhausted that I didn't even know what day it was as we made our way home. It wasn't until we left the hospital that the emotional dam finally broke and the tears started flowing. I was physically and emotionally drained for the next several days.

The following appointment our baby passed the fetal ultrasound but still had an unreactive NST. My blood pressure was even higher than before so I had to take a urine sample to test for protein just in case. Overall, the doctor was happy that we would make it to 34 weeks, which was another developmental milestone. He then stated that once we hit 34 weeks his threshold for allowing anything would dramatically go down and that we should be ready with our hospital bags. We started coming in three times a week for BPP, and the two appointments that followed were very similar – elevated blood pressure, non-reactive NST, and a passing fetal ultra-sound. Every day was exhausting and stressful. The baby's movements were starting to seem more sluggish, but since we passed another appointment, we assumed we would have a day in between to try and relax.

That night, as I was about to step out of the shower, I felt a huge gush of water. I looked down to see that my water had broken, except that there was bright red blood every-where. Through all of my research, I had heard many things about what your water breaking should look and smell like, but I hadn't ever heard anything about there being blood. Panic crashed over me as I instantly knew that something was wrong. I called my OB, who told us to come to the hospital right away, and we haphazardly gathered our things and headed off to the hospital. On the way I tried to research and understand what might have happened and came to the conclusion that it could be a placental abruption. The 27-mile drive seemed to take forever, and I hadn't felt the baby move at all. Relief rushed over me once I was hooked up to the fetal heart monitor and heard the baby's heartbeat. My baby was still ok. My contractions were starting to become uncomfortable, and the baby's heart was not tolerating them very well at all. It was 11:30 PM by that point, and the doctor told us we would be having the baby soon via C-section. Everything was happening very quickly, but for some reason I felt ready. The surgical team was amazing and made the entire situation very light and even had us laughing several times while everything was being prepped and I was getting my spinal. They even let us pick out the music we wanted to hear. Before we knew it, we heard our baby boy's cry. It was the most beautiful sound I had ever heard.

Our baby boy, Mason, was born on May 11 at 12:24 AM at just 3 pounds and 14 fourteen ounces. Come to find out, my placenta had detached and was the size of a very small hamburger patty. Our son was then taken to the NICU but surprisingly to everyone involved, came home with us when we were discharged from the hospital just four short days later at 3 pounds and 10 ounces! Our son has astounded us every day since and proven how much of a fighter he and all IUGR babies are. Mason is now eighteen months old, is on track developmentally, and has just made it onto the growth charts for a head circumference at twenty percent and height at seven percent. Our pediatrician is fully expecting him to hit the growth charts for his weight for his second birthday.

Questions and Medical Responses Raised by Colby's Story

1. What is a first-trimester screen?

   A first-trimester screen is several blood tests obtained from the pregnant mother in the first trimester of pregnancy. These tests evaluate for certain genetic conditions that can affect the pregnancy or baby.

2. What is a placental abruption?

   A placental abruption is separation of the placenta from the uterus before the baby is born. A placental abruption can be partial and small, slow and chronic, or very fast and severe. Usually a placental abruption is suspected when the amniotic fluid breaks and is found to be bloody or when vaginal bleeding is present, but the amniotic sac has not broken. In severe cases, a placental abruption can be life-threatening to the baby. Sometimes the cause of a placental abruption is known, such as after trauma to the mother's abdomen. Other times the reason for the placental abruption is not known.

3. What is concerning about the baby not moving?

    A baby who is not moving can be normal. This can occur when the baby is sleeping. However, it can also indicate that the fetus is not getting enough oxygen from the placenta, such as in the case of a placental abruption.

4. What is baby aspirin? Does it help with growth restriction?

    Baby aspirin is also known as low-dose aspirin. Some research studies show that low-dose aspirin can improve blood flow to the placenta in women who have or are at high risk for preeclampsia.

5. Does a high-protein diet help with growth restriction?

    Having a healthy diet is important to overall health of the mother and developing fetus. A high-protein diet may not help growth restriction, but it is also unlikely to hurt a developing fetus. Talk with your obstetrical provider before starting a diet during pregnancy.

6. What are PAPP-A levels?

PAPP-A is the abbreviation for "pregnancy-associated plasma protein-A." Low levels of PAPP-A are associated with stillbirth, growth restriction, preterm birth, and preeclampsia.

7. What is a normal placenta size?

Placentas normally grow during pregnancy, so the size of a normal placenta changes for each gestational age. Obstetricians and pathologists, who are physicians who specialize in making diagnoses from tissues taken from the body, use charts to determine whether a placenta is normal in size. At full term, the average placenta weighs around 500–600 grams, or 17–21 ounces, but healthy placentas can be smaller or larger than this average.

Family Story #5: Hilarie

I have had seven pregnancies, three of which ended in miscarriages. With my fifth pregnancy, baby was delivered April 16, 2010. He, like my other two full-term babies, was born 90–95% percentile for height and weight. I knew that I could grow big healthy babies when I stayed pregnant past twelve weeks. I was good at that.

In late December when I shared with Luke that I thought I was ready to have another baby, he was floored. He knew a miracle had happened. I had completely changed my heart and was willing to risk the possible difficulties for our baby girl.

When I went into my 20-week scan, I don't remember many specifics except that they requested that I do a repeat. They said that I was closer to 19 weeks, so they wanted to check things out more. Looking back, the doctor, not my regular OB but one of the MFM specialists, who I would get to know better when I was admitted to the hospital, may have mentioned something about Sophie measuring small. I am assuming that was the case. They probably already suspected she had IUGR but didn't want to unnecessarily scare me too early. That was August 16, 2017. My repeat scan was scheduled for September 6, 2017. I had no idea what whirlwind would await.

The morning of September 6, I woke up early and excited to see my baby again at our 9 AM scan. I went into this pregnancy exercising and eating healthier than I had my entire life. I felt great! I didn't have much nausea at all. But that all changed when I reached eleven weeks. I started feeling sick and unwell in general. I was close to the second trimester when energy is supposed to return, but it never did. I kept getting sicker and sicker. I didn't really notice that it was progressive and assumed I had some kind of late onset hyperemesis gravidarum. It had been twelve years since I had had it with Madeleine. We found out at twelve weeks we were indeed having our baby girl Sophie, and I assumed I just was sicker with baby girls. I had to cancel many of my obligations outside of home and work. And by July, I had to stop working because the sickness was so bad. By mid-August, I also started having chest pains which I just assumed were really bad gas pains. But none of the gas medications that were approved for pregnancy would even touch the pain. By the first part of September it was so painful that after driving for ten to fifteen minutes, I would have to pull over and readjust for a moment of relief in order to be able to drive ten more minutes. After the scan and ordered tests, I would learn that it was actually my liver shutting down from the early-onset severe preeclampsia I was experiencing. I don't want to get ahead of myself though.

I woke up early on the sixth to catch Luke before he left to go to the farm for work and asked Luke for a blessing. In my religion, men who hold the priesthood, which Luke did, could give blessings of comfort with the feelings and impressions coming from God through the priesthood holder. I had already asked for several during my pregnancy. And we had traditions that Luke would give our children blessings each year as they started school, and any other time of big change. In this blessing at 5:30 AM on September 6, the words or promise that stood out to me most was that Sophie would be born strong and healthy. I remember thinking that was odd, because I was only 22 weeks 5 days pregnant. I thought, ok that's good, but that won't be for another 16 weeks and a couple days, or so I thought.

I checked in for my scan at 9 AM. I was taken back, and my vitals were taken. My blood pressure was 180/90. I hadn't ever had hypertension, so I didn't know how high that was. My doctor was called immediately, and I could tell the worry present in the room. He ordered several labs and told me he'd follow up with me when he got the results. He called me at 4 PM that day and said that my liver enzymes were elevated and that my platelet count was low. I was also spilling protein in my urine. He ordered an ultrasound to look at my gallbladder and liver because of the pain I was experiencing. I went in the next morning and had the scan. He called back midday and said my gallbladder was fine but that my liver was not ok. He told me to come in first thing the next morning. Luke already had a work trip booked to go to Oregon to source his Christmas trees for that upcoming season. I assumed that worst case scenario I would be told to go on bed rest, and very worst case I would be admitted for hospital-monitored bed rest. I was nervous for the appointment, so I had my mom meet me at the hospital for the 8 AM appointment.

My doctor met me, still worried, and took my stats. My systolic blood pressure was still in the 180s. They did the ultrasound. They said that she may be small for gestational age but that the ultrasounds can be up to a pound off. They told me that they thought she weighed at least two pounds. My doctor sat me down and said, "You aren't going to like this, but we are admitting you to the hospital." I asked if I could go home and get any clothing or supplies, and he said no. I wrote a list for my mom to go and get.

They checked me into Labor and Delivery and started me on magnesium sulfate. As they had explained, my head did start to get fuzzy, and I felt like I was burning up. I still assumed that I would be spending the next several, hopefully at least ten weeks in the hospital while our baby Sophie continued her development. They were monitoring both of us. Within an hour, all of the MFM specialists in the hospital were in my room telling me that they were prepping me for a C-section. WHAT?!?! My husband had just arrived in Oregon, and … and … Sophie was just 23 weeks old that day.

The anesthesiologist came in and told me he was going to prep me for surgery and give me a spinal. I had had that with my two sons, so I was ok. He came back five minutes later and said he wanted to try an epidural. As soon as he placed it, my blood pressure dropped down to 160/80. The team decided that I could be given the choice to wait it out as long as we could or to deliver her then. Of course I wanted to give Sophie as much of a chance of survival as possible, so I said I wanted to wait. Some, if not most, of the team were upset and felt like I was risking both of our lives by waiting. The ones that were the most upset made certain that I was aware that at any moment they could override my choice if my blood pressure became too high. I was given the first of two steroid shots to help Sophie's lungs and to help keep my preeclampsia at bay. I miraculously was able to give her 48 hours. They were a rough 48 hours. I was in and out of consciousness at one point. My BP was elevated. The nurses told me they were surprised that I didn't have a seizure. I was hooked up to an arterial line, which was something most of the staff said they had never seen done before in labor and delivery.

But we gave her as much time as we could. We were told her chances of survival were low, but I had been promised she would be born strong and healthy. And that she was! The respiratory therapist said that in his 30 years of working with NICU infants, he had never seen a stronger, healthier 23-weeker. She was born in the second percentile. She weighed only 480 grams (just under 17 ounces). She was tiny, teeny tiny. My NICU team told me how shocked they were to see how small she was, but she was a fighter. She was strong and healthy, like God had promised!

Sophie continued to amaze the entire NICU staff. We were told that she would have rough days and that the stay would be a rollercoaster ride, but it wasn't. She passed all of the tests and made such great progress. I could see her every six hours for her cares. I tried to make every one that I possibly could. Sometimes, I would sneak peaks at her even at non-cares times. I LOVED being by her side. We were connected, and her fighting spirit was so big and so strong. All of her scans showed that her organs were healthy. Most surprisingly, she had no brain bleeds at all. I was told that that was unheard of. I was released from the hospital when Sophie was five days old but made the drive back two to three times a day to see her. I LOVED that time. I was pumping and producing good milk that she was tolerating well.

When she was ten days old, her teeny size presented its first major problem. It was time to remove the umbilical cord IV that they had been using for blood draws, but her veins were so tiny. It took six hours and ten attempts to place a PICC line. I was there for five of the hours. When they finally were able to place it in her head, I was allowed to come back and be with her. She was utterly exhausted. It killed me to not be able to hold my baby girl tight and kiss her sweet tiny head and soothe her with my love. They told me that because she was so tired and worn out that even what usually soothed her, like reading to her, could potentially stress her more. I left the hospital broken-hearted. I got in my car and bawled but came back for her next cares. She looked so much better. She was such a resilient fighter.

Then, on day thirteen, I was called at 5 AM and was told Sophie was struggling. This was our first time to experience a struggle with her. I tried to make it to rounds and was always told how well she was doing and what a miracle micro-preemie she was. But this morning, her first primary nurse that we had chosen found that the PICC line had broken. They did a scan, and she was struggling in many ways. I didn't realize in just how many ways. When I got there at 8:30 AM for her 9 AM cares, sweet Sophie was laid on her back, and her other primary nurse told me she had had a rough night. I read her two books and normally would pump in her room. She told me that because she was struggling so much that I should pump somewhere else. That was hard for me to hear, but I never wanted to jeopardize my Sophie's health for my selfish desires. While I was pumping, a nurse was sent to find me. She told me that the neonatologist wanted to talk to me. I got there, and she asked if Luke was around. He wasn't, and she suggested I call him to come as quickly as possible. The neonatologist who had been with her the twelve previous days was now off, and I met this doctor for the first time. It was a rough first meeting because she had to tell me the multitude of ways that Sophie was struggling. I told her that I truly believed that it was ok and that I had been told she would have hard times. I knew she would get better. The doctor looked at me with sympathy and said, "No, Sophie's body is giving up." I don't remember all the details after that, but I know that Luke showed up soon. I told him everything the doctor had told me. I think she also met with Luke, but I don't really remember. I just wanted a miracle. We had seen so many miracles with her. I asked the staff if there was another priesthood holder from our religion there, and they found one. Luke went to give her a blessing. I was waiting to hear him bless her with promises from God that she would heal and be made whole. Those never came. He was only able to bless her with comfort in the difficulties she was facing. I screamed in my head. She was our Sophie. We had waited and prayed for her for so long. I was ready to raise another infant, even if she had many delays and disabilities. But at 11 AM, her thirteen-year-old sister, Luke, and I were finally able to hold her as she took her last breaths and passed peacefully in our arms.

Questions and Medical Responses Raised by Hilarie's Story

1. Why did the PICC line break?

   Sophie was a very tiny baby, and her blood vessels were slightly larger than the size of a hair. The PICC line that had to be placed for her was also the size of a hair, so placing a PICC line was very challenging. PICC lines that are this small are more prone to breaking than larger PICC lines. However, Sophie's small size precluded placing a larger PICC line in her blood vessels.

2. Why did Sophie's body "give up"?

   Unfortunately, when a PICC line breaks, bacteria can get into the baby's body. A few bacteria can make premature babies sick quickly because their immune systems are weaker than a full-term baby's immune system. Further, growth-restricted babies' immune systems work less effectively than the immune systems of babies of average growth. Sophie's body most likely was struggling to fight the infection. Her little body was not able to do so effectively, even though she was receiving as much medical support as possible.

3. What is hyperemesis gravidarum?

   Hyperemesis gravidarum is a condition that causes severe nausea and vomiting in pregnant women. Some women require IV fluids and nutrition in addition to medications to treat nausea.

4. What is magnesium sulfate?

   Magnesium sulfate, often called "mag," is a medication given to women who are expected to deliver a preterm infant less than 32 weeks' gestation. Magnesium sulfate can improve the developmental outcomes for a baby. Magnesium sulfate also is given to prevent eclampsia in pregnant women, which is a severe form of preeclampsia that causes seizures.

Family Story #6: Meagan

Matilda is our "tiny but mighty baby." She is our eighth child. The first half of my pregnancy went great! At my 20-week ultrasound I found out that our baby was a girl and that she had all her body parts. She measured right on track. A month later, I did the routine glucose tolerance test and tested positive for gestational diabetes. In my previous pregnancies I never had gestational diabetes. The gestational diabetes might have been due to my older age, 43 years old, and weight. I was referred to a diabetes nutrition specialist to help me monitor my blood sugar and diet. I now had to eat protein with everything, watch my carbs, and check my blood sugar four to six times a day. I remember being very scared for our baby girl and hoping she would be okay. Nevertheless, I still enjoyed my pregnancy and was able to eat some good things. I was put on the medication, metformin. Because of the gestational diabetes they did an extra ultrasound to monitor the baby's measurements and to decide whether she would need to be delivered a week or two early.

I went into my ultrasound happy and feeling great. I was doing a great job of monitoring my blood sugar. The metformin and my diet were helping together. The ultrasound technician was checking me and was very positive while she was checking me. I asked her if the baby looked healthy and had all her parts still. She said she was. Then she was quiet, so I automatically thought our baby must be really big and asked her if the baby looked extra big due to my gestational diabetes. She said that the baby actually measured small for that point in the pregnancy. The technician told me one of the maternal fetal medicine doctors had to come look at things. At this point, I began to realize this was more serious than I thought. The doctor came in, looked at my ultrasound, and re-measured everything. I started getting very nervous. She showed me the ultrasound and told me that our baby was not growing as fast as she should. She was not sure when the decrease in growth started, so she recommended more frequent monitoring with non-stress tests done to watch her growth and heart rate.

This is when we first learned that our sweet baby girl was IUGR. I thought gestational diabetes was a scary diagnosis, but this was scarier. I had never heard of the term IUGR, so of course I looked it up online. It was pretty nerve-racking and shocking that our little baby was not growing. I had a lot of unanswered questions and was very worried. The things I read did not tell me much more than what the doctor told me. She was not growing as she should and therefore was small. She had to be monitored more closely. They could not give us an explanation why she wasn't growing.

My first non-stress tests before finding out my baby was IUGR went well. They would watch her heart rate, check amniotic fluid levels, and watch her growth. I sat in the bed, and they strapped a heartbeat monitor to my stomach. They found the heart rate and hooked it to a computer. We watched the heartbeat. Our baby did great for her first test. I was able to go home and breathe.

The second test was done five days after the ultrasound when we found out she was growth restricted. During the test, there were a few dips in our baby's heart rate. After the dips her heart rate went right back up, so the nurse said that it might be okay and that we would just watch me. Just to be safe after another dip in heart rate, she decided to get the doctor. The maternal fetal medicine doctor came in to check my results. When he came in there was another dip in heart rate. He looked at the readings of dips in heart rate and said that he was concerned. Then he said, "I think the baby needs to come out today." He did not want to take any chances. I had to text my husband at work. I told him that I was being prepped for an emergency C-section and that he should meet me at the hospital. Our baby girl was coming early, but we were at least grateful that we had made it to just over 34 weeks pregnant. Apparently in the NICU world, this is the magic number.

The C-section went great. Our "tiny but mighty" baby, Matilda, was born on January 12, 2018. She weighed 3 pounds 10 ounces and was indeed tiny. She cried right when she came out and could breathe great. She looked great except for her being very small. They brought her straight to the NICU. Because she was a preemie, she had to have an IV put in. Then she had a feeding tube put in and was kept warm.

Since Matilda was IUGR, the doctor sent in my placenta to be tested because they weren't sure what caused her to be IUGR. My doctor said that my placenta did not look good. The circulation did not look right, and the placenta was infarcted possibly. Matilda was breathing great and doing well in NICU. She was feisty when she started drinking the bottle. She was definitely mighty and strong in spirit. This really helped her thrive. Matilda stayed in the NICU for ten days. It was quite an emotional rollercoaster having Matilda in the NICU. It seemed like every day was a new day of ups and downs in her learning to drink out of a bottle and to be able to stop and take breaths on her own while eating. The NICU had to keep her body temperature regulated, make sure that she was eating enough, and keep an eye on her oxygen levels. And then we had to do another test to see if her IUGR was caused by anything else. Matilda had to have the cytomegalovirus (CMV) test next. CMV scared us the most because it causes hearing loss, liver problems, and calcium deposits in the brain. We had to wait 24 hours for the results. It was a long night of waiting and worrying with no sleep because we were so worried what the results would be for Matilda. We were relieved the results were negative. We felt blessed and so grateful. Eventually, the tests came back that my placenta had a clot in it. The clot was the most likely cause of Matilda's growth restriction.

Matilda continued to thrive in the NICU and was eating like a champ. She was breathing well and even passed her car seat test. She really wasn't gaining weight very fast and that worried us. The doctors said that she was ready to go home. At that point, she was only 3 pounds 11 ounces. She was tiny. I was very worried about taking her home to our other seven kids with germs floating around in the middle of respiratory syncytial virus (RSV) season. It scared me to take her home away from the doctors and nurses because she was so tiny due to her growth restriction. The label of IUGR made me extra worried to take her home. I was still trying to wrap my head around her being growth restricted and what it all meant. It was quite emotional for me and a scary time. I asked the doctor to let her stay another day but was denied because the insurance wouldn't pay for it if she was eating and breathing well. I was told weight wasn't an issue. She ultimately ended up being able to stay an extra two days because of a short breathing issue, which quickly resolved, but those two extra days were a help for me to mentally prepare to take care of an extra tiny baby. I hope that the NICU can be more aware of these babies and what their families go through during this time. Now Matilda is a healthy and spunky little girl.

She just turned two years old and is running around having fun with all her brothers and sisters. She is on the small side, but she is growing and doing very well! Matilda sure is "tiny but mighty."

Questions and Medical Responses Raised by Meagan's Story

1. What is RSV? What is RSV season?

   RSV is a common virus among children. Premature babies are particularly at risk for RSV. RSV, like many respiratory viruses, are more common in the wintertime. The RSV season is usually between November and April, but the exact timing varies each year.

2. What is a car seat test?

   A car seat test is a test to make sure that a baby has normal oxygen levels in the car seat before going home. This test usually is performed on babies who have required oxygen or who were born prematurely.

3. Why was Meagan scared to take Matilda home?

   It is normal for parents to feel a little afraid of taking a tiny baby home, particularly one who has been in the NICU. In the NICU, babies are hooked up to monitors and watched by specialized nurses and doctors 24/7. At home, parents do not have the same medical support as they had during their NICU stay. Not having the constant information from the monitors and NICU staff can make a parent feel that they are missing a critical piece of information about the health of their baby. Neonatologists are careful to monitor a baby in the hospital before deciding that it is safe to send a baby home.

CHAPTER 5

How Does Growth Restriction Impact Health in Childhood through Adulthood?

After the immediate newborn period, one of the biggest challenges for growth-restricted babies is to have a healthy rate of growth. We call this growth, "catch-up growth," because the baby is "catching up" to her peers who did not have growth restriction. How fast a baby should catch up is still hotly debated among physicians and researchers. The reason for this debate is because a baby who catches up in weight too quickly is somewhat more likely to have challenges with her metabolism, which may include obesity, high blood pressure, diabetes, high blood lipids, and high cholesterol in adulthood. For example, one research study shows that growth-restricted children with rapid catch-up growth between birth and two years of life had more fat around the organs in the abdomen than children who did not have catch-up growth by two years of life. However, while babies that catch up too slowly do not have as high of a chance of developing these metabolic challenges in adulthood, some studies suggest they are more likely to have problems with learning and cognition as they grow up. Unfortunately, we do not know yet what the optimal timing for achieving catch-up growth is, and it is possible that the optimal timing of catch-up growth may be different for every growth-restricted baby.

Fast catch-up growth, as mentioned above, can be associated with an increased chance of developing metabolic problems later in life, such as diabetes and obesity. Metabolic problems are health problems that affect how the body processes nutrition. The increased metabolic risks of rapid catch-up growth occur because the body is "reprogrammed" by the decreased delivery of nutrition before birth to hold on to calories. The body deposits the extra calories into the fat tissues, especially within the abdomen. These changes are a setup for problems with obesity and diabetes in the baby's future. Additionally, even though the weight and abdominal size of a child with a history of growth restriction may be the same as children without growth restriction, there is an increased risk of extra fat around the organs in the abdomen, more abdominal fat, and less muscle and bone. This situation can be especially challenging for physicians and parents. Growth-restricted children also can start to deposit fat in parts of the body where fat should not be stored, such as in the liver, muscles, bone marrow, and pancreas. The fat deposition can impede these organs from working normally. Abnormal levels of fat in these tissues can further increase the risk for lifelong metabolic problems, such as obesity.

Further complicating the potential metabolic health problems is that the brain can be reprogrammed by growth restriction to signal increased hunger. Leptin is a hormone in the body that tells the brain that the body is satisfied and no longer needs to eat. Leptin levels can be low in the blood of growth-restricted babies at birth. Low leptin levels may encourage growth-restricted babies to eat more. However, these low leptin levels do not always increase to normal levels in childhood. The brains of these growth-restricted children may not get the leptin signal from the body to stop eating, so these children may continue to eat more than their bodies need.

Before we can talk more about how the body and brain can be reprogrammed, we need to first cover the basics of how our genes allow our body and brain to function. Unless we have a problem with our genes or chromosomes, everyone has the same number of genes. We have approximately 20,000 genes in each of our cells, but we do not all look the same, think the same, or act the same. The reasons for these differences are that the information coded within each gene is slightly different for each person, and the environment in which we each grow and develop is different. For example, having different information coded within the genes for eye color allows one person to have brown eyes and another person to have green eyes. These genes do not change over time and are passed down from parent to child.

Our genes hold the information about who we are, but this information must be translated into a form that impacts how the body functions, such as telling the body to make brown or green colored eyes (**Figure 10**).

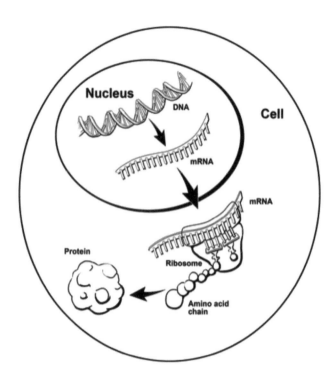

The normal process of translating genetic information into functional information. Genes are composed of DNA. A copy of the DNA of a gene is made. This copy is called mRNA. mRNA binds to a protein called a ribosome, which brings together specific amino acids to make a protein.

Figure 10

To translate information from a specific gene to a body function, the gene first makes a temporary copy of itself, called messenger ribonucleic acid (mRNA). mRNA contains the same information as the original gene but in a way that the body can use to translate into a function by making a protein. mRNA is translated by ribosomes into chains of amino acids that form proteins. Proteins are the workhorses of the body. Each protein carries out a specific function based on what the genes coded it to do. For example, one gene can code for a protein to make brown eyes, while another gene can code for a protein to make blonde hair.

Additionally, the protein produced by each gene can be turned up or down like a light bulb on a dimmer switch in a house. The many light switches in our house are like our genes. All the information in our genes is available, but only some of the information is used at a time, just as we do not turn on all of the lights in the house all the time. We choose which lights we want to have on depending on our needs. We can turn on lights in the kitchen when we need to cook and lights on in the office when we need to work. Further, we can choose to keep some lights on dim and others on fully bright. In the same way, our bodies can make a little bit of one protein and a lot of another, depending on our needs.

Reprogramming works like this: a baby who has growth restriction from an environmental or infectious cause has normal genes, but the baby needs to adapt to her environment of low nutrition and low oxygen to survive. A baby cannot change the information in her genes to allow her to hold on to the calories and oxygen that she gets. To adapt, she must change the extent to which specific genes are expressed. For example, in response to not having enough nutrition, a growth-restricted baby can increase the amount of mRNA that forms proteins that bind sugar in the blood and bring it into the body's cells to be used as energy (**Figure 11**).

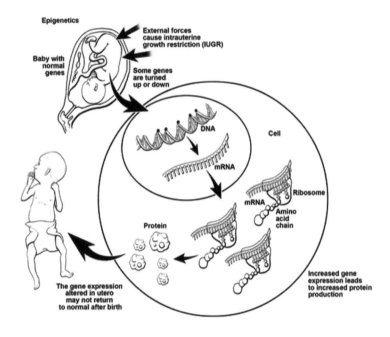

*The process of adapting to a poor environment by changing
how many proteins are made from certain genes.*

Figure 11

Reprogramming is a way to adapt to a stressful environment. It is a very useful skill for survival. But after birth, sometimes the reprogramming does not go back to normal. Even though the growth-restricted baby is getting enough nutrition after birth, the level of the sugar binding proteins may not return to normal, and the baby's body may continue to bring extra sugar into cells. In our light–switch analogy, this process of reprogramming is like leaving the lights on fully bright in the kitchen all of the time, even though we do not need those lights to be on. The extra sugar brought into cells gets stored in the body as fat. Over time, the excess fat predisposes a person to metabolic health problems like obesity and diabetes. Researchers are actively trying to find the key to restore the normal function of our genes, or in our analogy, how to give us access to all of the dimmer light switches in the house again. However, researchers are just starting to understand how the genes got stuck in the first place.

While fast catch-up growth increases the chance of having metabolic health problems later in life, avoiding catch-up growth altogether is not the answer. Growth-restricted babies who do not have catch-up growth tend to remain shorter than those who have catch-up growth. Babies who do not have catch-up growth also can have problems with thinking, learning, social interactions, and fine motor skills like handwriting. In some small studies, babies who did not have catch-up growth by nine months after birth were more likely to have problems with development. Though the recommended timing of when catch-up growth needs to occur is different in various studies, most studies agree that catch- up growth needs to happen to minimize developmental problems.

About ten percent of growth-restricted babies will remain short by the time they are two years old. Growth hormone supplementation has been recommended for these children who remain significantly shorter than expected. Pediatric endocrinologists, who are pediatricians who specialize in disorders of the endocrine system, may recommend treatment with growth hormone for growth-restricted children who are too short at two years old. The definition of too short depends on the biological parents' heights, whether the child is a boy or a girl, and the age of the child.

Growth-restricted children are more likely to have learning difficulties, which can impair a child's school performance. Approximately one in every three children who were growth restricted at birth have learning difficulties. Learning difficulties may be more common in children who were symmetrically growth restricted compared to children who were asymmetrically growth restricted. Usually these learning difficulties are mild. The brain of growth-restricted fetuses physically develops differently than that of others, which may increase the chances of learning difficulties and impaired school performance. Some studies also suggest that growth-restricted children are two to five times more likely to have behavioral problems, attention deficits, or hyperactivity, such as attention deficit disorder (ADD) or attention deficit hyperactivity disorder (ADHD). The risks for these behavioral challenges may be increased more by the underlying reason for growth restriction, such as maternal substance use, rather than the growth restriction itself. Some research studies associate growth restriction with a five to ten times increased chance of having mood disorders, such as anxiety and depression; however, this link is still controversial.

Growth-restricted children also are more likely than others to get infections from viruses and bacteria. The smaller the baby is at birth, the greater the risk for infections in childhood. Viral and bacterial infections are common in children. The impact of growth restriction on getting an infection is relatively small, around a ten percent increase in risk. Overall, growth restriction increases the risk of infections the most during the first year of life, but there is still an increased risk of infections for the first ten years of life. Growth restriction can alter how the immune system works and decreases the number of certain infection-fighting white blood cells and proteins. The type of infections seen in average-sized and growth-restricted children usually are the same, but the growth-restricted children may get more of these common infections. Good nutrition after birth and throughout childhood is associated with fewer infections in children who were growth restricted at birth.

General recommendations from researchers on growth restriction recommend that pediatricians follow these children more closely. These recommendations include checking blood pressure every year, keeping a close eye on patterns of growth that would suggest changes in metabolism leading to health conditions, such as obesity and diabetes, and being more aggressive about checking and treating conditions, such as high blood lipids and diabetes. Your pediatrician will discuss the risks and benefits of each of these interventions with you based on your child's specific health conditions.

The metabolic and developmental health problems that growth-restricted children can have may continue into adulthood. An adult who was growth restricted at birth generally is four to five times more likely to have obesity, diabetes, high blood pressure, high blood lipids, and high cholesterol. These adults are more likely to have heart attacks and strokes. Growth restriction also alters how the kidneys function, which further increases the chances of developing high blood pressure. Even if an adult who was growth restricted at birth does not have obesity, she is more likely to have abnormal fat deposits in the tissues in her body such as in the muscles and liver, which can cause higher blood lipids, high blood pressure, and diabetes. Growth restriction also alters how the bones develop and increases the risk of bone fractures and osteoporosis, which is characterized by weakened bones. Each of these health conditions are often treatable with lifestyle modifications and medications. Therefore, it is important for adults who were growth restricted to follow closely with their physician.

Growth restriction also can increase the risk of infertility in adults. While most adults who were growth restricted at birth are able to have children without significant difficulty, they are more likely to have difficulty getting pregnant. Once pregnant, women who were themselves growth restricted at birth are more likely to have certain health conditions. Women who were growth restricted at birth are more likely to have diabetes and obesity in adulthood and are more likely to have these conditions during pregnancy, too. Diabetes and obesity are two health conditions that can complicate pregnancy and the health of the baby. Therefore, it is important for these women to be evaluated by their obstetrical provider throughout pregnancy.

Health risks from growth restriction can be passed on to the next generation. Studies have found that the reprogramming effect can persist and be passed on from parent to child. A person who was herself growth restricted at birth can pass on a similar pattern of reprogrammed genes, and thus health risks, to her own child, even though her child may not be growth restricted. Obesity and diabetes in pregnant mothers increase the risk of having large infants at birth, which is called large for gestational age. Despite the different appearance of large for gestational-age and growth-restricted babies after birth, large for gestational-age infants and infants whose mothers have diabetes undergo a similar process of reprogramming and have similar childhood and adulthood health risks as growth-restricted infants.

What Parents Can Do

A balanced approach to nutrition and close monitoring of your child's growth and health, in close partnership with your child's pediatrician, are probably the best ways to minimize risks of both metabolic and developmental problems. Most severely growth-restricted babies will need extra calories after birth for a few months or longer, though mildly growth-restricted babies often do not need extra calories. Extra calories are given to babies by mixing a fortifier into mother's milk or by providing a higher calorie formula. Mother's milk and regular formula contain approximately 19 or 20 calories per ounce. Extra calories are given usually as either 22 or 24 calories per ounce. Mothers can breastfeed still and are encouraged to do so. If your baby's physician determines that the baby needs extra calories, you can add a couple of bottles of higher calorie formula into the feeding schedule each day and breastfeed the rest of the time, or you can pump breastmilk and add powdered formula to your breastmilk. Other options include encouraging your baby to eat more frequently, to eat greater amounts, and to eat for longer amounts of time. Extra calories are needed sometimes for a few months or sometimes for a few years, depending on how your baby's growth is overall. Your physician will help you decide what the ideal feeding is for your baby.

If you notice that your baby is gaining weight quickly, talk to your doctor. In babies who were not growth restricted, periods of rapid weight gain are normal. Periods of rapid weight gain in growth-restricted babies can be normal but should be monitored closely to help minimize the potential long-term health risks.

As your child grows and develops into adulthood, teach your child the benefits of healthy eating habits and exercise. While eating well and exercising are important to everyone, they are especially important for growth-restricted people.

Studies show that parent bonding and interaction improves their baby's development. Encouraging and supporting your child's education may significantly improve their school performance. Activities such as reading to your child, teaching your child, and playing with your child can improve their intelligence and social interactions. If your child seems to be falling behind in school, talk to your child's teacher and to your child's physician to see if additional therapies may help.

Family Story #7: Eliana

My name is Eliana. I am 20 years old and am currently a junior in college. I was born in Guatemala City, Guatemala and was adopted when I was five months old. I was born just under six pounds as an IUGR baby. From what I know, my birth mother was malnourished and under severe amounts of stress during her pregnancy with me. Ultimately these factors affected my size as a baby and possibly caused other mental health issues that were detected further down the road. She was a single mother of two kids from a previous relationship and was incredibly poor. Most likely she was working extremely long hours during the day.

Although I don't have much knowledge on what exactly it means to be an IUGR baby, I am discovering things about my own personal health and medical history that lead me to wonder if being a small baby had anything to do with them. While growing up, I was a pretty healthy kid besides frequent ear infections. My real health struggles came around middle school when I was diagnosed with mono for the first time. Throughout my middle school and early high school years, I had both Epstein-Barr virus (EBV) and CMV mono. My liver and spleen were heavily affected by these viruses. I also had nine different staph and MRSA infections. After years of dealing with extreme fatigue from the mono, I still couldn't seem to regain my energy or full strength. Throughout my life, I have worked with many different doctors and treatments, including Western, Ayurvedic, Chinese, homeopathic, and herbal. Each new form of medicine contributed positively to my health and my knowledge of my body as a whole. Although I know more about my body now, there will always be information that will remain a mystery given that I have no access to family history due to my adoption.

Ever since I was little, I always worried. Some worries were reasonable, and some weren't. Growing up in the suburbs of Chicago, I always felt the need to protect myself and my family and knew when something didn't feel right.

However, I had no idea that this type of anxiety wasn't "normal." As I got older, I started going to a therapist where I was diagnosed with both general anxiety disorder and depression. Things started to make more sense about why and how much I worry. I was given medicine, which helped for a while. In middle school, my grandparents died, which caused me to fall into a severe depression. I was beginning to self-harm. I developed an eating disorder, and I was suicidal. Everything seemed like it was falling apart, and that was when I began taking medication for my depression. I have always been "depressed" in a way due to knowing that my birth mother had to give me up for adoption but was never this depressed. I barely finished middle school. There was still concern that I might not be able to continue on to high school. Eventually, medicine really helped with both my anxiety and depression. I was able to see a very small light at the end of the tunnel. Moving from middle school to high school was a very exciting experience, and knowing that I would be able to move on helped me to pull through and gave me some hope.

My anxiety and depression still exist; however, I am in a much better place and have them under control through the use of both Western and homeopathic medicines and herbs. My attention deficit hyperactivity disorder (ADHD), however, was not discovered until I was a junior in high school. Gradually, it became harder for me to focus. All of this combined with my anxiety made it very hard for me to keep up with schoolwork. Eventually, learning testing was done, and I was diagnosed with ADHD. I have been taking medicine for the past four years, which has helped tremendously. I was able to get the help that I needed through my high school and college, which is amazing.

Questions and Medical Responses Raised by Eliana's Story

1. What are EBV and CMV mono?

   Mono is short for mononucleosis, which is an infectious disease characterized by extreme fatigue, sore throat, rash, and body aches. Both EBV and CMV can cause mononucleosis. Growth restriction impairs the way the body's immune system functions and can increase the risk of infections such as mononucleosis.

2. What are staph and MRSA infections?

   Staph is short for staphylococcus, which is a family of bacteria that can cause infections. MRSA stands for methicillin-resistant Staphylococcus aureus, which is a particular type of staphylococcus bacteria resistant to the antibiotic, methicillin, and other similar antibiotics. Growth restriction impairs the way the body's immune system functions and can increase the risk of infections such as bacterial infections.

3. What is ADHD?

   People with ADHD have difficulty concentrating on a task. Lower cognitive scores have been seen in school-age children with growth restriction, but research studies are still conflicting regarding whether ADHD is specifically associated with growth restriction.

4.   Are Eliana's health conditions caused by growth restriction?

It is hard to say what contribution Eliana's growth restriction has on her specific health conditions. Growth restriction has been linked to increased infections, including viruses and bacteria. The link between growth restriction and learning difficulties in childhood is well-established. Research studies conflict on how much of a role growth restriction plays in a person developing ADHD, anxiety, and depression.

Family Story #8: Laura

My first child, my son, was born a few days after the 40-week mark. He weighed 7 pounds 6 ounces. About a year and a half later I became pregnant with my second child, my daughter Lydia. At an ultrasound around 30 weeks, my OB indicated that the baby was "measuring small" but hanging steady around 24th percentile in size. There were no signs that she was not getting enough fluid or blood or that there were placenta problems. My OB said I was "growing well a small baby," but he did recommend that I drink a protein shake daily and have another ultrasound in three weeks.

At the 33-week ultrasound, my OB noticed that the baby had fallen off the normal growth curve, from the 24th percentile around week 30 to the tenth percentile at week 33. He recommended weekly ultrasounds at a MFM office. He also tested for toxoplasmosis, which was negative. He tested for no other viruses due to, as he told me, a high rate of false positives when testing for other viruses.

Part of me felt relieved to have a weekly ultrasound at the MFM office to check on the baby. At week 35, she was in the fourth percentile. It was at one of those MFM visits that a doctor first mentioned a suspected diagnosis of "IUGR." I didn't understand what that meant, other than that the baby was small and should receive more careful monitoring to check that she was growing ok. When I looked up IUGR on the internet to try to understand what might be causing IUGR or what it might mean for the baby's health, the search results were pretty scary. Most things I read discussed chromosomal problems or viruses as probable causes. Some were associated with serious health complications and negative outcomes. Despite asking my OB and the MFM office staff questions, I wasn't able to learn much about what having IUGR might mean for my baby's health.

At one visit to the MFM office, the doctor suggested that I pack a bag and be ready to go to the hospital and deliver right away if an ultrasound found that the baby wasn't doing well. I remember calling my parents and crying when I explained what the doctor had said. My parents later told me that it was that tearful phone call when they realized that this IUGR diagnosis might be something serious.

My husband and I tried to keep a positive attitude. We also wondered if the baby was just small because we are on the small side. The doctors advised us to just wait and see after the baby was born. My doctor indicated that the baby likely may need to go to the NICU but might not need to stay for long.

The doctors recommended that I deliver on the day the baby hit the 37-week mark, suspecting that the environment in the uterus was keeping the baby from reaching her growing potential. In week 36, as the delivery date approached, I was put on bed rest and had two ultrasounds.

Lydia was born on the first day of the 37th week as planned, weighing 5 pounds 7 ounces. She passed all the standard infant tests. I was so relieved she was healthy! None of the doctors or nurses mentioned IUGR. I asked about it a few times, but I got the sense that because Lydia appeared to be healthy, the doctors did not feel a need to address the IUGR or investigate it.

Lydia stayed in my room throughout the hospital stay. She had no troubles with breathing, blood sugar levels, or jaundice. She was very tired the first few days and didn't have much energy to suck, so for a day or so we fed her expressed milk with a dropper. Due to her small size, before she was allowed to come home, the hospital required her to pass a "car seat test." She needed to sit in a car seat and maintain good vital signs for a period of time (about 45 minutes, I think). This test was performed out of our sight, and we heard from a nurse that it had taken Lydia two tries to pass.

I mentioned the IUGR diagnosis at her infant appointments with our pediatrician. He said Lydia seemed healthy, and nothing suggested complications from IUGR. Lydia continued to meet all developmental milestones, and I didn't think about IUGR again until she was seven months old. During a routine pediatrician visit, our pediatrician recommended adding a teaspoon of high-fat coconut oil or olive oil to her food, since she was in the seventh percentile in weight. We supplemented her solid foods with coconut oil for several months.

And that is basically all! I have hardly thought about the IUGR diagnosis since. I am ever grateful that Lydia is healthy and that she didn't need to spend time in the NICU or require special medical interventions when she was born. I wonder how many other IUGR diagnoses end up being ultimately as uneventful as our experience.

Lydia is now a happy seven-year-old. She has not had any health problems that the pediatrician has attributed to IUGR. She remains quite petite. She has consistently been at less than the tenth percentile for height and weight and was at the first percentile for both during her seven-year well visit. After the initial recommendation to supplement Lydia's food with coconut oil when she was a baby, our pediatrician has not recommended any health or diet interventions based on her small size. Lydia is energetic, kind, smart, and bold—tiny and definitely mighty!

Questions and Medical Responses Raised by Laura's Story

1. How can we know whether a baby has IUGR or is just small? Is it possible a baby could both have IUGR and be genetically predisposed to being small?

   Small babies are sometimes perfectly healthy. Not every baby who is small is also growth restricted. Sometimes it can be very difficult for doctors to know if a baby is small because they are genetically predisposed to being small or if they are small because they are growth restricted. Unfortunately, there is not a test to say that a baby definitely has growth restriction. However, sometimes babies have features that indicate that the baby has growth restriction. These features may include a particularly low body weight with a head size that is only slightly smaller than expected or not enough fat stores under the skin, which makes the baby look skinny. Additionally, a baby can be both genetically predisposed to being small and growth restricted.

2. When is it appropriate to supplement a baby or toddler's food with coconut oil or another high-fat food?

   Growth-restricted babies are watched closely for appropriate weight gain. Doctors plot a baby's growth on growth charts to know if a baby's weight gain is appropriate. Doctors will usually recommend supplementation by either feeding the baby a special formula with extra calories or by adding formula to pumped mother's milk. Growth-restricted babies who have slow catch-up growth are more likely to have delays in development later in life, so having catch-up growth is important. Toddlers and children are also at risk of not having good weight gain. Doctors often will recommend supplementing the diet of toddlers and children with a high-fat food if their weight gain is not following the normal curves on growth charts.

3. If doctors do not seem inclined to investigate the potential cause of IUGR either during pregnancy or after birth, should parents nevertheless advocate for it?

    Researchers are continuing to evaluate why growth restriction happens and what we can do to treat it. Because new information is being published frequently, it can be difficult for doctors to keep up with the most recent information about growth restriction. For example, it is only recently that CMV was found to cause growth restriction, and treatment for CMV is now available to give to newborns. Testing is not always necessary, particularly if the baby is doing well and the doctor is not sure whether the baby has growth restriction. However, it is always ok to ask your doctor if testing for causes of growth restriction is appropriate.

4. How often are babies with IUGR born essentially healthy? How often do they avoid spending time in the NICU?

    Because each hospital has different guidelines for when a baby needs to go to the NICU, it is hard to say how many growth-restricted babies go to the NICU. Some hospitals require that a baby go to the NICU for a low blood sugar that requires NG tube feedings. Other hospitals require that a baby go to the NICU only if NG tube feedings are unable to keep the baby's blood sugar normal and the baby needs IV fluids. Most babies with growth restriction do quite well and do not need to spend time in the NICU. Fortunately, most often these tiny but mighty babies lead full and healthy lives.

5. Are babies who are SGA more likely to have health problems even if they are not diagnosed with growth restriction?

    SGA babies who are not diagnosed with growth restriction are usually healthy. However, SGA babies are at increased risk for a few health issues after birth. For example, SGA babies are more likely to have low blood sugar than babies that are average weight for gestational age, and most hospitals have policies in place to monitor the blood sugar levels of an SGA baby.

Conclusion

I hope that this book has helped you better understand the diagnosis of growth restriction and feel more prepared to embrace your child and what lies ahead. I encourage you to ask your health care provider questions, connect with IUGR communities online or in person, and seek out resources for your particular situation (see Appendix 1 for an initial list of suggestions).

One of the contributors to this book, Colby, sums up well the parting thoughts that I hope you take from this book:

> "Our OB couldn't have described it better. IUGR babies are nature's miracles. Because of all the stress that they are exposed to while in utero, it makes them stronger than a baby who is just born early. I often look back in disbelief on the emotional rollercoaster we experienced but mostly on how far we all have come. We couldn't have made it through such a stressful and sometimes seemingly hopeless journey without all of the love and support from our families, friends, and IUGR support groups, as well as the amazing doctors and nurses we got

to know along the way. It is definitely true what everyone says. IUGR babies are tiny but mighty, and we couldn't be more in love."

Resources for Families

1. *Understanding the NICU: What Parents of Preemies and Other Hospitalized Newborns Need to Know*, by Zaichkin, Weiner, and Loren. 2017.

   a. This is an easy-to-understand guide to help parents understand NICU technology and terminology.

2. *Intrauterine Growth Restriction: Aetiology and Management.*

   a. This is a very dense reference intended for physicians, but this resource has a great amount of detail for parents who want a lot of information and who are medically savvy.

3. There are numerous support groups online and in person. Some of these groups can be found through:

   a. The website associated with this book: www.tinybutmightybaby.com

   b. Websites such as www.magicfoundation.org and www.fetalhealthfoundation.org

c. Facebook

d. NICU social worker

e. NICU parent-to-parent groups

Tenth Percentile Weight for Each Gestational Age

The following chart is an estimate of the tenth percentile birth weight for gestational age for girls and boys (**Figure 12**). Each population, country, and race has small differences in the weights at each gestational age, and the numbers are frequently revised. Further, because few babies are born at the earliest gestational ages, we do not have as robust information about what the tenth percentile for weight is for these babies. Therefore, this table is only an estimate. In some cases, these estimated weights may be off by several ounces or more. Data for this table were based on data from the American Academy of Pediatrics and the Fenton growth curves. In this table, the average weight is for both boys and girls and is equivalent to the 50th percentile. The 50th percentile means that half of babies are born weighing more than the weight listed, and half of babies are born weighing less than the amount listed.

Gestational age (weeks)	SGA girl (grams)	SGA boy (grams)	Average (grams)
22	415	432	508
23	441	467	584
24	473	509	657
25	515	561	746
26	570	624	851
27	642	700	966
28	735	790	1096
29	850	896	1240
30	900	980	1338
31	1050	1130	1578
32	1200	1300	1790
33	1400	1500	2018
34	1620	1730	2255
35	1840	1950	2493
36	2060	2180	2726
37	2290	2400	2947
38	2480	2600	3156
39	2650	2800	3360
40	2820	3000	3568
41	2980	3200	3785
42	3150	3400	4014

Estimate of the tenth percentile birth weight for gestational age for girls and boys in grams.

Figure 12

Gestational age (weeks)	SGA girl (pounds)	SGA boy (pounds)	Average (pounds)
22	14.6 oz	15.3 oz	1 lb 1.9 oz
23	15.6 oz	1 lb 0.5 oz	1 lb 4.6 oz
24	1 lb 0.7 oz	1 lb 1.9 oz	1 lb 7.2 oz
25	1 lb 2.1 oz	1 lb 3.8 oz	1 lb 10.3 oz
26	1 lb 4.1 oz	1 lb 6 oz	1 lb 14 oz
27	1 lb 6.7 oz	1 lb 8.9 oz	2 lbs 2.1 oz
28	1 lb 9.9 oz	1 lb 11.9 oz	2 lbs 6.7 oz
29	1 lb 14 oz	1 lb 15.6 oz	2 lbs 11.7 oz
30	1 lb 15.7 oz	2 lbs 2.7 oz	2 lbs 15.2 oz
31	2 lbs 5 oz	2 lbs 7.9 oz	3 lbs 7.7 oz
32	2 lbs 10.3 oz	2 lbs 13.9 oz	3 lbs 15 oz
33	3 lbs 1.4 oz	3 lbs 4.9 oz	4 lbs 7.2 oz
34	3 lbs 9.1 oz	3 lbs 13 oz	4 lbs 15.5 oz
35	4 lbs 0.9 oz	4 lbs 4.8 oz	5 lbs 7.9 oz
36	4 lbs 8.7 oz	4 lbs 12.9 oz	6 lbs 0.1 oz
37	5 lbs 0.8 oz	5 lbs 4.7 oz	6 lbs 7.9 oz
38	5 lbs 7.5 oz	5 lbs 11.7 oz	6 lbs 15.3 oz
39	5 lbs 13.5 oz	6 lbs 2.8 oz	7 lbs 6.5 oz
40	6 lbs 3.5 oz	6 lbs 9.8 oz	7 lbs 13.7 oz
41	6 lbs 9.1 oz	7 lbs 0.9 oz	8 lbs 5.5 oz
42	6 lbs 15.1 oz	7 lbs 7.9 oz	8 lbs 13.6 oz

Estimate of the tenth percentile birth weight for gestational age for girls and boys in pounds.

Figure 13

IUGR and NICU Glossary

Advanced practice registered nurse: a nurse who has received additional specialized training in the care of premature and sick newborns and who functions similarly to a physician

APS: antiphospholipid syndrome. APS is a medical condition of the immune system.

BPD: bronchopulmonary dysplasia. BPD is a condition of breathing problems due to prematurity. BPD is another term for CLD.

BPP: biophysical profile. A BPP is a series of ultrasound measurements that includes the non-stress test information. The five tests in a BPP are an NST, breathing movements, body movements, muscle tone, and amniotic fluid levels.

Chromosome: a large collection of genes

CLD: chronic lung disease (of prematurity). CLD is a condition of breathing problems due to prematurity. CLD is another term for BPD.

CMV: cytomegalovirus. CMV is a virus that can cause developmental delays and hearing impairment in the baby, most often if the mother gets CMV during pregnancy.

CPAP: continuous positive airway pressure. CPAP is a type of breathing support through the nose that babies sometimes need in the newborn intensive care unit.

CTG: cardiotocography. CTG is another term for a non-stress test, which is a tracing of the fetal heart rate.

Developmental delay: a condition in which a child does not meet developmental milestones

Diabetes: a condition of impaired secretion of or response to insulin resulting in high blood sugar

Early term: between 37 0/7 and 38 6/7 weeks' gestation

EBV: Epstein-Barr virus. EBV is a virus that can cause a condition called mononucleosis.

Extreme prematurity: less than 28 weeks' gestation

Extremely low birth weight (ELBW): less than 1000 grams birth weight (2 pounds 3 ounces)

Fetus: an unborn baby

FGR: fetal growth restriction, another term used to define a fetus that is smaller than expected

Genes: inheritable genetic information passed from parent to child

Gestation: the period of time between conception and birth

Growth restriction: another term used to define a fetus that is smaller than expected

Hypertension: high blood pressure

Infant: a baby that is between 30 days of life and one year of life

Inflammation: a condition where tissue becomes hot, red, swollen, and painful, possibly due to an infection

Intravenous (IV) fluids: a solution usually containing sugar and electrolytes that is given directly into a vein

Isolette or incubator: a specific bed designed for premature newborns to provide humidity and heat to the baby

IUGR: Intrauterine growth restriction, the term used to define a fetus that is smaller than expected

IV: intravenous. An IV is a thin tube that is placed inside a vein to give medications or fluids to a patient.

Large for gestational age (LGA): greater than 90th percentile for gestational age

Late preterm: between 34 0/7 and 36 6/7 weeks' gestation

Low birth weight (LBW): less than 2500 grams birth weight (5 pounds 8 ounces)

MFM: maternal fetal medicine. A MFM physician is a doctor who specializes in high-risk pregnancies. A MFM doctor is also known as a perinatologist.

NEC: necrotizing enterocolitis. NEC is an infection of the intestines that can affect premature newborns.

Neonatal nurse: a nurse who takes care of premature and sick newborns

Neonatal nurse practitioner: a nurse who has received additional specialized training in the care of premature and sick newborns and who functions similarly to a physician

Neonatologist: a physician who specializes in the care of premature and sick newborns

Newborn: a baby between the time of birth and the first 30 days of life

Newborn intensive care unit (NICU): the location in a hospital where premature or sick newborns receive specialized care

NST: non-stress test. An NST is a tracing of the fetal heart rate.

Nursery: the location in a hospital where healthy newborns receive routine care

Obesity: a body mass index of at least 30

Overweight: a body mass index between 25 and 30

Pediatrician: a physician who specializes in the care of healthy or mildly ill newborns and children

Perinatologist: a physician who specializes in the care of high-risk pregnancies

Pharmacist: a medical professional who specializes in the dispensing of medications

PICC line: peripherally inserted central catheter. A PICC line is a type of intravenous (IV) line that is longer inside the body than a regular IV.

Placenta: the organ that develops during pregnancy, filters nutrients and oxygen from the mother's blood to the fetus, and filters fetal waste products back to the mother

Preterm: less than 37 weeks' gestation

Respiratory therapist: a medical professional who specializes in providing therapies to the lungs

ROP: retinopathy of prematurity. Retinopathy of prematurity is a condition unique to developing eyes in preterm infants.

RSV: respiratory syncytial virus. RSV is a virus that can cause coughing and difficulty breathing.

Small for gestational age (SGA): less than the tenth percentile for gestational age

SNS: supplemental nursing system. SNS is a way to feed a baby with extra formula or milk while the baby is working on breastfeeding.

Step-down or transitional nursery: the location in a hospital where babies who previously had required NICU care can continue recovering with specialized care

Term: between 39 0/7 and 41 6/7 weeks' gestation

Trimester: one-third of pregnancy, approximately three months

Uterus: the organ in the female body that allows for the conception, growth, and development of a fetus

Ventilator: a medical device that provides oxygen and pressure to the lungs and helps the lungs get rid of waste gas

Very low birth weight (VLBW): less than 1500 grams birth weight (3 pounds 4 ounces)

About the Author

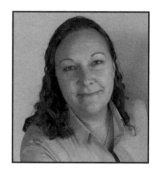

ERIN ZINKHAN, MD is a neonatologist, which is a physician who is an expert in caring for tiny and sick babies. After completion of her medical school training at the University of Texas Southwestern Medical School, she completed Pediatrics Residency and Neonatology Fellowship at the University of Utah. Dr. Zinkhan had a productive academic career before joining private practice in Neonatology.

Dr. Zinkhan is one of the world's leading experts in intrauterine growth restriction. She is a doctor who cares for growth-restricted, premature, and sick babies in the newborn intensive-care unit. She dedicated her research to unveiling the reasons why growth-restricted babies are more likely to have health problems throughout life. She has published multiple research articles and presented her research at international conferences to further the medical community's understanding of growth restriction. Now, she also focuses her time on educating the general public about growth restriction. She started the blog, Tiny But Mighty

Baby (www.tinybutmightybaby.com), to provide a resource for families to learn more about growth restriction and stay up-to-date on research advances. Proceeds from this book are donated to a foundation started by Dr. Zinkhan to fund research that discovers ways to improve the lives of people with growth restriction.